# RUNNER'S WORLD TRAINING JOURNAL FOR BEGINNERS

Sheila Anderson

*Name*

shelovesart@hotmail.com

*Phone/E-mail*

Oct 17, 2014 –

*Journal Dates*

sanderson91592@marykay.com

858-336-9503

# RUNNER'S WORLD®
# TRAINING JOURNAL FOR BEGINNERS

## 52 WEEKS OF

- MOTIVATION
- TRAINING TIPS
- NUTRITION ADVICE
- AND MUCH MORE

FOR RUNNERS WHO ARE JUST STARTING OUT

BY THE EDITORS OF RUNNER'S WORLD®

RODALE.

Rodale books may be purchased for business or promotional use or for special sales. For information, please write to:
Special Markets Department,
Rodale Inc., 733 Third Avenue, New York, NY 10017



Printed in the United States of America
Rodale Inc. makes every effort to use acid-free ♾, recycled paper ♻.

Excerpts by coach and exercise physiologist Susan Paul, *Runner's World* "For Beginners Only" columnist appear on pages 43, 57, 71, 85, 99, 113, 127, and 141

Book design by Elizabeth Neal

Library of Congress Cataloging-in-Publication Data is on file with the publisher.
ISBN 978–1–60961–539–0 paperback

Distributed to the trade by Macmillan

2 4 6 8 10 9 7 5 3 1 paperback

RODALE.

We inspire and enable people to improve their lives and the world around them.
rodalebooks.com

# CONTENTS

# INTRODUCTION

**FIRST I WANT TO CONGRATULATE YOU.** If you've picked up this journal, you've heeded the call to get moving.

Maybe that call has been whispering to you for years and grew louder each time you drove by someone running down the street or caught a glimpse of the old gym shoes gathering dust in the back of your closet. Or maybe that call was a little less ethereal—like doctors' orders or a blunt piece of unsolicited advice from a loved one. It doesn't matter, really. What matters most is that you listen to the call to run and have mustered the courage to start.

You won't regret it, I assure you.

Studies have shown that exercise is medicine, and that it will vastly improve the quality of your life and even help you live longer. A regular workout routine (150 minutes per week, which is about 30 minutes five times per week)—and running in particular—has health benefits that extend well beyond any pill a doctor could prescribe.

Running can help prevent obesity, type 2 diabetes, heart disease, high blood pressure, stroke, some cancers, and a host of other unpleasant conditions. It will lower blood pressure and cholesterol, increase energy, and improve depression and anxiety. If you're older, being fit will lower your risk of falling, mitigate age-related cognitive decline, and improve your quality of life. If you're overweight, it will help you shed pounds. If you've already lost weight, exercise will help you keep it off better than diet alone.

Sure, at first it's not going to be pretty. Or pleasant. As nice as it would be if we discovered our inner Olympian immediately upon taking our first steps and were instantly transformed into the most graceful and fit *Runner's World* cover-worthy versions of ourselves, for the vast majority of us, it just doesn't happen that way.

The first few times out, there's a good chance that working out will feel downright uncomfortable. There will be lots of "D'ohs!" "Oofs!" "Eeks!" "Ouches!" and "Oy veys!" There will be mornings when the alarm sounds and you feel like you have to pry your eyes open with a crowbar. The bones may creak; the muscles may cry; I assure you there will be lots of sweating, swearing, blisters, and smelly clothing.

But there will many more positive returns that keep you coming back, despite all this. You may discover beautiful vistas in your own backyard, you may sow lifelong friendships and have adventures that you wouldn't have otherwise. And if you start any run conservatively enough, there will be days when you feel like you're gliding effortlessly, and like you were *born* to run. And after you finish, you will get a sense of accomplishment and boost of confidence that you can ride all day long.

Mark Twain famously said, "I can live for 2 months on a good compliment," and I have found the same to be true from a good run. It doesn't matter if it's 1 mile or it's 10 miles. But as soon as I finish, I feel confident, strong, hopeful, and more capable of taking on whatever chaos the day may bring. I feel like a much better version of myself than the one I was before I hit the road.

Celebrate your successes in this training journal. On days when you're feeling low and unmotivated, look back on the miles you've logged as a reminder of how much you've accomplished and how good running can feel, and when you have setbacks—everyone has them, even elites—you should record them too. Reviewing those and seeing how much you've overcome—whether it's an injury or the very strong urge to sleep in—will boost your confidence and remind you that you're stronger than you think you are, more powerful than you know.

The real magic, after all, is how running transforms you on the inside. Pushing your body and mind farther than they've gone before—over and again—on the roads has a powerful impact on every other area of your work and family life. You gain an appetite for adventures and the courage to make them happen. You go from believing that you can't to wondering whether you can.

This log is a valuable training tool to help you get started on an exercise routine, stick with it, and get fitter. As you write the story of your own running life, consult some of the other sections of the book for *Runner's World*'s best tips on training, nutrition, and injury prevention.

Be sure to read the stories of inspiring new runners who got up the courage to take their first steps and just kept going, despite embarrassment, fear, setbacks, injuries, and their own deepest doubts about whether they could do it. We also included some of the most frequently asked questions from beginners like you and answers from Susan Paul, an exercise physiologist and running coach, who has worked with thousands of runners as program manager for the Orlando Track Shack Foundation. And she's helped scores more *Runner's World* readers through her weekly column "For Beginners Only," on runnersworld.com. We hope that all the tools in this training journal—and these moving stories—will give you the courage and the know-how to take this journey yourself.

***—Jennifer Van Allen***
Special Projects Editor
*Runner's World*

# HOW TO USE THIS JOURNAL

This training journal is more than just a mileage log; it's a valuable tool that can help you build your fitness and stay motivated and injury free. Take good notes and look for patterns. For instance, you may notice that your back aches when you run on the roads, but you feel great on days when you run on the trail. Feeling bored and unmotivated to get out the door? You might look at your log and see that you've been doing the same neighborhood loop for months in a row, and it's time to mix it up. All this information can help you design the best running routine for you to stay happy, healthy, and safe. Above all, seeing all the miles and minutes pile up—and we encourage you to total your mileage each week and month for a confidence boost—can help you stay motivated to run on days when it's tough to get going. Below is some information that you might want to include.

- Daily or weekly goal
- Mode of exercise (run, elliptical, swim, bike, etc.)
- Distance (in miles or kilometers)
- Workout duration
- Weather conditions
- Time of workout (this can influence how you feel)
- Route and terrain (hills, treadmill, track, trail)
- How you feel before, during, and after the run
- Shoes and gear used
- Music, books, or podcasts you listened to
- Interesting things you saw along the way
- Notes about the people you ran with

# TRAINING

Walking, and running, are two of the least expensive and most convenient ways to get fit, lose weight, reduce stress, and improve your quality of life.

Before you start, take these steps to get into the habit of regular exercise and lay a solid foundation for your running life.

**GET CHECKED.** If you're over 40, or have a family history of heart disease or other health problems, see a doctor before you start a regular exercise program.

**WALK, THEN RUN.** Though some people dismiss *walk* as a four-letter word, it is the most effective way to develop the fitness you need to start running comfortably—without injury. Walking puts your legs and arms through the same general range of motion as running, but without the same impact on your bones and joints. The walk should be brisk—not a race walk, but not a window-shopping walk either, says Steven Blair, professor of exercise science and epidemiology and biostatistics at the University of South Carolina.

**START SMALL.** And build slowly. The idea of starting an exercise routine can seem daunting. It doesn't have to be. Begin with a 15-minute walk. Feeling good? The next day, do it again. If you're feeling strong, add 5 or 10 more minutes. Work up to 35 minutes by the end of the week.

**GET GOOD GEAR.** Resist the temptation to just wear any old pair of tennis shoes for your workouts. Worn-out or ill-fitting shoes are one of the most common causes of injury. Go to a specialty running shop, where someone can help you find a pair that offers the fit and support you need. "There's no magical shoe that makes running easier, but a bad shoe will ruin your running," says Bruce Wilk, a Miami-based physical therapist, coach, and owner of The Runner's High shop. So don't shop by price, fashion appeal, or bold promises. While you're at the store, get clothing made with lightweight, technical materials like Drymax or SmartWool that wick sweat away from your skin so you stay cool in the summer, warm in the winter, and dry even when it's wet outside. Anything cotton will soak up moisture like a sponge and keep you cold.

**MAKE THE TIME.** Establish a workout routine that blends well into the rhythm of your daily life. Figure out what times of day are most convenient to work out and find a variety of safe, traffic-free routes that you can take on a regular basis. Find the time of day when running is nonnegotiable. For many people that's first thing in the morning, when no meetings are scheduled and the kids are still in bed. And make sure that you have cleared enough time to work out so that it doesn't jam up your day.

**COUNT YOUR CALORIES.** Track your intake with a food journal (you can use a pen and paper or try one of the many free Web sites and apps on the market). Studies have shown that those who keep food diaries—who are also reading nutrition labels and becoming aware of portions—lose more weight than those who don't.

**BUILD YOUR OWN SUPPORT SYSTEM.** Enlist a buddy for your first outing to the gym or trail, or try a group workout or a class. Research shows that connecting with others—whether it's a person, an online forum, or a workout group—increases your chances of sticking with an exercise routine. And remember that everyone feels self-conscious at first. "We get so caught up in the anxiety and fear of being negatively evaluated by others," says Christy Greenleaf, a professor of kinesiology at the University of Wisconsin. "But the reality is that most of the time other people are way more concerned about themselves."

**SNEAK IN SMALL ACTIVITIES.** Take a few minutes of your lunch break to walk the office halls; park at the back of the lot; take the stairs instead of an elevator; and set a timer to chime every hour to remind you to get up and walk around, says running coach Janet Hamilton, MA, CSCS, an exercise physiologist at Running Strong in Atlanta. Even standing rather than sitting at your desk will help. Studies have shown that standing at your desk during an 8-hour workday will burn 163 more calories than sitting.

**GET A PLAN.** While you may not feel like you need a schedule for working out, having a training plan will help keep you on track to meet your goals and ensure that you build up your workout time gradually enough that you don't get injured. Plus, crossing off each workout as you complete it will give you a sense of accomplishment and confidence. See page 150 for our Start Walking plan.

# NUTRITION

## How to Eat like a Runner

When you start exercising regularly, you might have to revamp some of your everyday eating habits in order to feel your best while you're working out and avoid unwanted bathroom stops. Here's how to reshape your diet to help support your new running life, from Pamela Nisevich Bede, author of the "Fuel School" column on runnersworld.com.

**GO ON EMPTY (SOMETIMES).** What you eat before you hit the road or the gym all depends on when you're exercising and what kind of workout you're planning. Many people can't eat and digest food before a workout, especially if it's in the early morning. For an easy workout of 1 hour or less, going without food probably won't do you any harm. (Just make sure you're staying hydrated.) But for any event that's longer or more intense, preworkout fuel is critical.

**KEEP IT SIMPLE.** What's the perfect preworkout meal? Familiar foods that are easy on your system, low in fat and fiber, and high in carbs will boost your energy without upsetting your stomach.

**TIME IT RIGHT.** When it comes to fueling your workout, timing is everything. In general, the bigger the meal the more time you'll need to digest. Each person is different, but for most people, it's best to eat at least 30 minutes before heading out so you don't have GI distress when you're on the road.

**DRINK UP.** Hydration is important, and not just when you're exercising. Fluids regulate body temperature, move waste from your body, ensure that your joints are adequately lubricated, and help flush out the damaged cells that can lead to inflammation. And proper hydration can help control cravings. While there's no set recommendation for daily fluid intake, a good rule of thumb is to aim to drink about half of your body weight in ounces each day. (So if you weigh 150 pounds, drink 75 ounces of water.) Stick with calorie-free beverages like water. And you don't have to just guzzle. Fruits and vegetables can also help you stay hydrated. Plus they're packed with antioxidants, which boost muscle recovery and immunity.

**GET THE BALANCE RIGHT.** Even if you're not exercising with a goal of losing weight, you still need the right mix of foods and nutrients to feel energized on your runs and to stay injury free. About 55 percent of your daily calories should come from carbohydrates, 25 percent should come from protein, and another 15 to 20 percent should come from unsaturated fats. But there's no need to start carrying around a calculator. At each meal, simply devote half of your plate to carbs, one-quarter of your plate to protein, and slightly less than a quarter to healthy fats.

**TAKE OUT THE TRASH.** Grocery shop with a "clean kitchen" in mind. Limit the high-sugar, high-fat foods you toss in your cart; if they're not in the house, you won't be tempted to eat them. Stock your fridge with fruits, veggies, and whole grains, so they'll be there when mealtime rolls around. Those foods will keep you feeling good when you're working out, plus they'll keep your heart healthy, your cholesterol low, and your blood sugar stable.

# 10 Tricks to Lose Weight Fast

You can shed weight quickly, depending on how much you have to lose and how focused you remain. Oftentimes simple, easy changes can help you see results right away. That said, patience is an important part of the successful weight-loss formula. The pounds didn't get packed on overnight; it's going to take some time to establish healthy eating and exercise habits and shed the not-so-healthy ones. Here are some tips from Pamela Nisevich Bede, author of the "Fuel School" column on runnersworld.com.

**1. DO SOME DETECTIVE WORK.** Identify the most likely culprits for the unwanted weight. Are fried or sugary foods too tough to resist? Is it hard to avoid noshing whenever free food is nearby? Are you too tired and busy to cook healthy meals? The answers to these questions may lead you to your first best steps.

**2. GET MOVING.** It's difficult to lose weight by just cutting calories. Research shows that reducing calorie intake through diet *and* exercise is the most effective way to shed unwanted pounds and keep them off. It's ideal to develop a regular exercise routine of three or four times a week. (See page 150 for the Start Walking plan, which can help you get into the habit of regular exercise and stick with it.)

**3. PLAN AHEAD.** Everyone has weak moments—situations where it's tough to make healthy choices. Make a list of those occasions where your diet tends to take a detour. No healthy lunch options at work? Pack your own. Devour everything in the fridge in the 10 minutes after you walk in from work? Snack on the way home and precook a dinner that you can reheat right when you get home. If you go off the rails late at night, think of another activity far from the kitchen that helps you relax. Try a book, a shower, a call to a friend, a hot bath, or a fun movie.

**4. FILL UP ON FRUITS AND VEGGIES.** You *can* eat large portions without loading up on calories—as long as you're eating fruits and vegetables. Compared with other foods, produce is low in calories and high in nutrients, fiber, and water, all of which will help you lose weight without being hungry. Produce is also a good source of unprocessed carbohydrates, so it can help keep you energized when you're on the road. Fill half your plate at every meal with fruits and vegetables. Fill the other half with whole grains and lean protein—lean cuts of meat, beans, tofu, or low-fat dairy—to keep you feeling fuller for longer.

**5. DON'T DRINK YOUR CALORIES.** Stick to calorie-free beverages like water or hot tea. A 20-ounce soda can pack 240 calories and 65 grams of sugar. If you love specialty drinks, choose a smaller size with fat-free or low-fat milk and skip the whipped cream and syrups.

**6. DON'T DO ANYTHING DRASTIC.** It's difficult to feel bad about your body or have a burning desire to be thinner. Everyone wants to get thin now. But crash diets that promise to help you do that—by limiting you to a small group of foods, drastically reducing your calorie intake, or requiring you to buy certain engineered foods—won't work. Even if you lose weight fast, you'll likely regain the weight and then some. If you want the weight loss to last for life, you need to make changes that you can sustain for life.

**7. SET SMART CALORIE TARGETS.** Eating three meals each day keeps your metabolism revved, keeps you burning calories, and prevents you from getting so ravenously hungry that you eventually eat everything that's not tied down. If you restrict your meals to fewer than three per day, you'll be more likely to go overboard as soon as anything edible is within arm's reach.

- Women: Aim for 300 to 500 calories a meal.
- Men: Aim for 400 to 600 calories a meal.
- Women and men: Aim for a 100- to 200-calorie snack.

**8. KEEP TRACK.** Studies show that people who track the calories they consume lose weight and keep it off more than those who don't. And there's good reason. When you have to track your calories, you see the sources of empty calories that are low on nutrients. In order to accurately track calories, you have to measure out portions—another practice that's proven to aid weight loss.

**9. DO NOT MAKE WEIGHT THE ONLY MEASURE OF SUCCESS.** Even as you get fitter, you may not see results on the scale. Keep in mind: Muscle weighs more than fat, and hydration, hormones, time of day, and other factors can all have an impact on the numbers on the scale. Are your pants getting looser? Are you getting more compliments? Do you have more energy? What about your blood pressure, cholesterol, and other markers of chronic disease? Which way are they moving? Those factors matter too.

**10. JUST PRACTICE; DON'T TRY TO BE PERFECT.** It's okay to indulge on occasion; one extra treat will not doom your diet. When you do go overboard, try not to wallow in guilt or anxiety about it. You can't control the past; all you can control is the choice you make right now. Work in enough foods that feel like rewards on a regular basis so that you don't feel deprived and primed to binge. Remember, it takes time, effort, and practice to form new healthy eating habits.

# INJURY PREVENTION

It's much easier to prevent an injury than to come back from one. The tips below can keep you on the road, and off the sidelines, so you can reach your fitness goals.

**1. AVOID THE TERRIBLE TOOS.** Doing too much, too soon, too fast is the number-one cause of running injuries. The body needs time to adapt to increases in mileage or speed. Muscles and joints need recovery time so they can handle more demands. If you rush that process, you could break down rather than build up. So be the tortoise, not the hare. Increase your weekly and monthly running totals gradually. Follow the 10 percent rule: Build your weekly mileage by no more than 10 percent per week. So if you run 10 miles the first week, run 11 miles the second week, about 12 miles the third week, and so on. There may be times when even a 10 percent increase proves too much. Use the 10 percent rule as a guideline, but realize that it might be too aggressive for you.

**2. LISTEN TO YOUR BODY.** Most running injuries don't just come out of nowhere and blindside you. Usually, there are warning signs—aches, soreness, and persistent pain. It's up to you to heed these signs. If you don't, you could hurt something else as you try to change your gait to compensate for the pain.

**3. GET GOOD SHOES.** Running shoes have changed a lot over the years, and there's a dizzying variety of models, brands, and types to choose from. There are even minimalist shoes designed to mimic barefoot running (although there's no scientific evidence that forgoing shoes decreases injury risk).

There's no single best shoe for every runner—your goal is to find the one that offers the best support and fit for *your* unique anatomy and biomechanics. Don't buy a shoe just because it's the cheapest, because it "looks fast," or because it matches your favorite workout gear. You should replace your shoes every 300 to 500 miles. Note the date that you bought your shoes in your training log so that later you'll know when it's time for a change. And when it's time to buy, visit a specialty running store—the staff there will ask you lots of questions, watch you walk or run, and take other steps to help you find the right shoe.

**4. TAKE GOOD NOTES.** This training journal can be a valuable tool in your efforts to stay safe and injury free. Take some time after each workout to jot down notes in this journal about what you did and how you felt. Look for patterns. For instance, you may notice that your knees ache when you run on consecutive days, but you feel great when you rest in between running days. This will help you determine the best routine for you. Plus, it will help get you out the door when the going gets tough. You can draw confidence from seeing all the miles pile up. And the next workout doesn't seem as daunting when you see how much you've already accomplished.

**5. CROSS-TRAIN.** Running is hard on your body, there's no doubt about it. So experts agree that most runners can benefit from cross-training activities to help improve muscle balance and stay injury free. Swimming, cycling, elliptical training, and rowing will burn a lot of calories and boost your aerobic fitness.

# Stay Safe on the Road

Take these precautions to protect yourself when you're walking and running outside.

**LEAVE WORD.** Tell somebody or leave a note at home about where you plan to go and how long you plan to be out. That way your loved ones will know to come look for you if needed.

**IDENTIFY YOURSELF.** Run with proper ID and carry a cell phone with emergency contacts taped to its back.

**PRETEND YOU'RE INVISIBLE.** Don't assume a driver sees you. In fact, imagine that a driver *can't* see you, and behave accordingly.

**FACE TRAFFIC.** It's easier to see, and react to, oncoming cars. And cars will see you more clearly too.

**BE SEEN.** Wear high-visibility, brightly colored clothing. When out near or after sunset, reflective materials are a must. (If you don't own reflective clothing, a lightweight reflective vest is a great option.) And use a headlamp or handheld light so you can see where you're going, and drivers can see you. The light should have a bright LED (drivers see blinking red as a hazard).

**UNPLUG YOUR EARS.** Avoid using iPods or wearing headphones—you need to be able to hear approaching vehicles. If you do use headphones, run with the volume low and just one earbud in so you can hear approaching vehicles.

**MIND YOUR MANNERS!** At a stop sign or light, wait for the driver to wave you through—then acknowledge with your own polite wave. That acknowledgment will make the driver feel more inclined to do it again for the next walker or runner. Use hand signals (as you would on a bicycle) to show which way you plan to turn.

# SHOES

If you want to stay healthy, fit, and injury free, invest in a good pair of running shoes. Worn-out or ill-fitting shoes are a leading cause of injury.

Follow these tips to make sure you get the pair that you need.

**DON'T SKIMP.** It may feel like a lot to spend up to $120 on a pair of running shoes, but the investment is worth it. Consider this: Whatever your new shoes cost, it is likely less than the money you'd spend seeing the doctor because you got hurt. (Not to mention less time consuming and less stressful!)

**SEE THE EXPERTS.** It's best to go to a specialty running shop (not a big-box or department store) where a salesperson can watch you run and help you select a pair of shoes that offer your feet the support they need.

**SIZE YOURSELF UP.** You may think you know your size, but it's best to get your feet measured each time you buy new shoes. Your feet change over time, and one model's fit can be drastically different from another's. Many people end up getting a running shoe that's a half size larger than their street shoes. The extra room allows your foot to flex and your toes to move forward with each stride. When you're standing with both shoes on, make sure you have at least a thumbnail's space between the tip of the shoe and the end of your longest toe. Try shoes on both feet and take them for a test run around the shop, on a treadmill, or on the sidewalk.

**BRING WHAT YOU'VE BEEN WEARING.** When you go shopping, take along the shoes, socks, and any inserts that you've been using. That way you can make a realistic evaluation of how well the new shoe will fit your feet.

**KEEP UP THE ROTATION.** Shoes should be replaced every 300 to 500 miles. Keep track of the date that you bought them in your training log.

**DON'T BE A TRENDSETTER.** It's easy to get wooed by a bargain-basement price, shoes that "look fast," or a promise to cure an injury or help you lose weight. But there is no one best shoe. There is only one shoe that offers your feet the unique support and fit you need. Try on as many different models and pairs as possible. And what about those minimalist shoes designed to mimic barefoot running? There's no scientific evidence that these shoes decrease injury risk. When you're just starting out, stick with traditional shoes.

Use the form below to record the date you bought your shoes in this log, so you'll know when it's time to replace them.

## SHOE NAME Asics

Date purchased: 10/17

Price: ____

Where you bought it: Sports Auth

Shoe size: 11

Foot size (measured—yes? no?): yes

Date you started using this shoe: ____

Date you retired this shoe: ____

Miles of use: ____

Notes: ____

## SHOE NAME ____

Date purchased: ____

Price: ____

Where you bought it: ____

Shoe size: ____

Foot size (measured—yes? no?): ____

Date you started using this shoe: ____

Date you retired this shoe: ____

Miles of use: ____

Notes: ____

## SHOE NAME ______________________________

Date purchased: _______________

Price: _____________________

Where you bought it: _________________

Shoe size:________________

Foot size (measured—yes? no?): __________

Date you started using this shoe: ________

Date you retired this shoe: _________

Miles of use: _________

Notes:____________________________________________

______________________________________________________

______________________________________________________

## SHOE NAME ______________________________

Date purchased: _______________

Price: _____________________

Where you bought it: _________________

Shoe size:________________

Foot size (measured—yes? no?): __________

Date you started using this shoe: ________

Date you retired this shoe: _________

Miles of use: _________

Notes: ___________________________________________

______________________________________________________

______________________________________________________

## SHOE NAME ______________________________

Date purchased: ______________

Price: ____________________

Where you bought it: ________________

Shoe size:_______________

Foot size (measured—yes? no?): __________

Date you started using this shoe: ________

Date you retired this shoe: _________

Miles of use: _________

Notes: ________________________________________

________________________________________________

________________________________________________

## SHOE NAME ______________________________

Date purchased: ______________

Price: ____________________

Where you bought it: ________________

Shoe size:_______________

Foot size (measured—yes? no?): __________

Date you started using this shoe: ________

Date you retired this shoe: _________

Miles of use: _________

Notes: ________________________________________

________________________________________________

________________________________________________

## SHOE NAME ______________________

Date purchased: ____________

Price: ________________

Where you bought it: ____________

Shoe size:____________

Foot size (measured—yes? no?): ________

Date you started using this shoe: ______

Date you retired this shoe: _______

Miles of use: _______

Notes: ______________________________

______________________________________

______________________________________

## SHOE NAME ______________________

Date purchased: ____________

Price: ________________

Where you bought it: ____________

Shoe size:____________

Foot size (measured—yes? no?): ________

Date you started using this shoe: ______

Date you retired this shoe: _______

Miles of use: _______

Notes: ______________________________

______________________________________

______________________________________

# TRAINING JOURNAL

 WEEK 1 WEEK OF 10/13 TO 10/19

## NUTRITION

At each meal, about half of your calories should come from healthy complex carbohydrates like fruits, vegetables, and whole grains. About one quarter of your calories should come from heart-healthy unsaturated fats like avocados, nuts, seeds, and olive oil. And the remainder of your calories should come from sources of lean protein like soy, fish, lean poultry, eggs, and beans.

"It's empowering to be able to do something you never thought was possible. And it carries over into work and relationships and everything else in real life. Now, I don't view anything as undoable. Nothing is off the table. That doesn't make it free, or easy. But now I have the confidence to know that if I'm willing to put in the work, there's nothing that can't be done. Running really showed me that."

—**ANDY AUBIN**, runner, Hatboro, Pennsylvania, runnersworld.com/andy-aubin

**MONDAY** 10/13

Route: Lake Miramar

Distance: 5 miles Time: 1:23:57

NOTES: first 5 miles!!

Cross-training:

**TUESDAY** 14

Route:

Distance: Time:

NOTES:

Cross-training:

**WEDNESDAY** 15

Route:

Distance: Time:

NOTES:

Cross-training:

**THURSDAY** 16

Route: River Walk

Distance: 3.02 Time: 52:40

NOTES: ☺

Cross-training:

**FRIDAY** 17

Route:

Distance: 6 miles Time:

NOTES:

Cross-training:

18

## SATURDAY

Route: Rest

Distance: Time:

NOTES:

Cross-training:

19

## SUNDAY

3mi Run

Route: Torrey Pines Hike

Distance: 6 miles Time:

NOTES:

Cross-training:
w/ BGR

## NOTES

WK 3/12 Build a Base!
WK GOAL = 17 miles.

WEEKLY MILEAGE TOTAL:

TOTAL MILEAGE TO DATE:

### INJURY

Get your feet measured each time you buy new shoes. Your feet change over time, and one model's fit can be drastically different from another's. Many people end up getting a running shoe that's a half size larger than their street shoes. The extra room allows your foot to flex and your toes to move forward with each stride. When you're standing with both shoes on, make sure you have at least a thumbnail's space between the tip of the shoe and the end of your longest toe.

### TRAINING

Take short strides. Keep your elbows flexed at 90 degrees and keep your hands relaxed, as if you were holding a piece of paper between your thumb and pointer finger. Stand and look straight ahead at the horizon; avoid looking down at your feet.

 GOAL 21 miles Nike+ WK 4/12 *

WEEK 2 WEEK OF 10/20 TO 10/26

## NUTRITION

For most people, a wide variety of factors lead them to pack on unwanted pounds. Take the time to identify what the issues are for you. Are fried or sugary foods too tough to resist? Are you too busy to cook healthy meals? Or do emotions—like boredom, anxiety, nervousness, and depression—send you straight to the fridge? If intense emotions are driving you to eat, use alternate routes that will offer relief without derailing your weight-loss goals. You might reach out to a friend, get more sleep, or sink into the distraction of a good book or movie.

*Build strength

"There is one thing exercise fosters everyone can use: the feeling of being glad to be alive. Exercise makes you happier."

—**GABRIELLE REECE**, former professional volleyball player and author of *My Foot Is Too Big for This Glass Slipper*

20 **MONDAY**

Route:

Distance: 3 mi Time:

NOTES:

Cross-training:

21 **TUESDAY**

Route: 3.8 mi

Distance: Time:

NOTES:

Cross-training:

22 **WEDNESDAY**

Route:

Distance: Time:

NOTES:

Cross-training:

23 **THURSDAY**

Route: 3 mi

Distance: Time:

NOTES:

Cross-training:

24 **FRIDAY**

Route: 8 miles :)

Distance: Time:

NOTES:

Cross-training:

25 **SATURDAY**

Route:

Distance: Rest Time:

NOTES:

Cross-training:

26 **SUNDAY**

Route:

Distance: 4 miles Time:

NOTES: Build Endurance 5/12 wk. = 24 miles GOAL

Cross-training:

**NOTES**

**WEEKLY MILEAGE TOTAL:**

**TOTAL MILEAGE TO DATE:**

## INJURY

Before beginning any new exercise regimen, it is important to consult with your primary care physician. It's especially important if you're over 40 or have a family history of heart disease or other health problems.

## TRAINING

Start each workout with 3 to 5 minutes of walking or easy running to warm up. This gives your muscles, bones, and joints a chance to loosen up; it gradually and gently brings up your heart rate and makes it easier to get into the rhythm you want to sustain so you can run—and finish—feeling exhilarated and energized enough to go longer, and excited to set out for your next workout.

WEEK 3 WEEK OF 10/27 TO 11/1

## NUTRITION

The most effective way to lose weight is to cut calories while also boosting your calorie burn through regular exercise. But avoid slashing too many calories too soon; that could cause your energy levels to take a nosedive and make your workouts feel even tougher. Start by trying to consume 300 fewer calories per day. With the other calories you burn through exercise, you can expect to lose a half pound to 1 pound per week.

27
### MONDAY

Route:

Distance: 6 Time:

NOTES:

Cross-training:

28
### TUESDAY

Route:

Distance: 3 Time:

NOTES:

Cross-training:

29
### WEDNESDAY

Route:

Distance: Time:

NOTES:

Cross-training:

30
### THURSDAY

Route:

Distance: 3 Time:

NOTES:

Cross-training:

31
### FRIDAY

Route:

Distance: 8 m. Time:

NOTES:

Cross-training:

> "There's no magical shoe that makes running easier, but a bad shoe will ruin your running."
>
> —**BRUCE WILK,** Miami-based physical therapist, coach, and owner of The Runner's High shop

Nov 1

## SATURDAY

Route:

Distance: Rest

Time:

NOTES:

Cross-training:

2

## SUNDAY

Route:

Distance: 4 miles

Time:

NOTES:

Cross-training:

## NOTES

WEEKLY MILEAGE TOTAL:

TOTAL MILEAGE TO DATE:

## INJURY

In the winter, check the wind chill before you head out. That's a measure of how cold it really feels when you're outside. As the wind grows stronger, it feels much colder than the air temperature.

## TRAINING

Walking is the easiest way to develop the fitness you need to run down the road. Walking puts your legs and arms through the same general range of motion as running, but without the same impact on your bones and joints, and without the same risk of getting hurt. Plus it gives you an opportunity to explore convenient, safe, traffic-free routes, which will become superimportant as you get into a routine.

## NUTRITION

Hydration is important, and not just when you're exercising. If you hydrate throughout the day, you don't have to worry about gulping down fluids just before a workout, which could upset your stomach on the road. While there's no set recommendation for daily fluid intake, it's good to aim to drink about half of your body weight in ounces each day. (So if you weigh 150 pounds, drink 75 ounces.) It's best to stick with calorie-free beverages like water to avoid packing on unwanted pounds.

"The first mile is always the hardest. And that's true whether it's your first run or you're out on a 10-mile run. Just get past that point. It always feels better after the first mile. It's not going to get easier, but every day you get stronger and better."

—**TARA CUSLIDGE-STAIANO,** runner, Stockton, California, runnersworld.com/tara-cuslidge-staiano

### MONDAY

Route:

Distance: Time:

NOTES:

Cross-training:

### TUESDAY

Route:

Distance: Time:

NOTES:

Cross-training:

### WEDNESDAY

Route:

Distance: Time:

NOTES:

Cross-training:

### THURSDAY

Route:

Distance: Time:

NOTES:

Cross-training:

### FRIDAY

Route:

Distance: Time:

NOTES:

Cross-training:

## SATURDAY

Route:

Distance: Time:

NOTES:

Cross-training:

## SUNDAY

Route:

Distance: Time:

NOTES:

Cross-training:

## NOTES

WEEKLY MILEAGE TOTAL:

TOTAL MILEAGE TO DATE:

## INJURY

Your main goal is to get fit without getting hurt. Going too far too fast, before your body is ready is one of the most common causes of injuries like shin splints, IT band syndrome, and runner's knee, which sideline many people. You can stay injury free by gradually building up the time you spend walking and running, increasing the time by no more than 10 percent from week to week.

## TRAINING

A few pieces of high-quality shorts, tops, and pants, will keep you comfortable while you're working out. Get clothing made with lightweight, technical materials like Drymax and SmartWool, which wick sweat away from your skin so you stay cool in the summer, warm in the winter, and dry even when it's wet outside. Avoid wearing cotton; it will soak up moisture, cause chafing, and keep you cold.

## NUTRITION

Don't know which foods are derailing your diet? Check out one of the online calorie-tracking sites or smartphone apps to learn more about what you eat. No time to cook a healthy meal? Precook a week's worth of dinners on weekends.

"Don't let your frustration today keep you from getting out there tomorrow, because tomorrow, you may just break through that time or distance barrier. But you'd never know that if you quit when things are hard."

—ANDREA "ANDI" BALL, runner, Elkridge, Maryland, runnersworld.com/andi-ball

### MONDAY
Route:

Distance: Time:

NOTES:

Cross-training:

### TUESDAY
Route:

Distance: Time:

NOTES:

Cross-training:

### WEDNESDAY
Route:

Distance: Time:

NOTES:

Cross-training:

### THURSDAY
Route:

Distance: Time:

NOTES:

Cross-training:

### FRIDAY
Route:

Distance: Time:

NOTES:

Cross-training:

## SATURDAY

Route:

Distance: Time:

NOTES:

Cross-training:

## SUNDAY

Route:

Distance: Time:

NOTES:

Cross-training:

## NOTES

WEEKLY MILEAGE TOTAL:

TOTAL MILEAGE TO DATE:

### INJURY

It's best to do strength training after a short run, where you finish feeling strong. It's best to leave rest days for rest. But if you're only running 3 days per week, strength training on a rest day or cross-training day is fine.

### TRAINING

Be as active as you can in your work and family life. The extra calories you burn will aid your weight-loss efforts and make your workouts feel easier. Climb the stairs of your office building before your lunch break or take a walk after you've eaten. Even standing rather than sitting at your desk will help.

WEEK 6 WEEK OF ______ TO ______

## NUTRITION

It's best not to drink your calories. Stick to calorie-free beverages like water or hot tea. A 20-ounce soda can pack 240 calories and 65 grams of sugar. Even a 16-ounce hot chocolate with fat-free milk can have up to 360 calories. If you love specialty coffee drinks, choose a smaller size with fat-free or low-fat milk and skip the whipped cream and syrups.

"Now I am doing things without breathing hard that would have killed me just a year ago. Being able to get so much more done and having the energy to do it is amazing. I thought that by running all the time, I would just be worn out and not want to do anything. But it's just the opposite. I can do more now than ever."

—**MATT TANNER,** runner, Vail, Arizona, runnersworld.com/matt-tanner

### MONDAY

Route:

Distance: Time:

NOTES:

Cross-training:

### TUESDAY

Route:

Distance: Time:

NOTES:

Cross-training:

### WEDNESDAY

Route:

Distance: Time:

NOTES:

Cross-training:

### THURSDAY

Route:

Distance: Time:

NOTES:

Cross-training:

### FRIDAY

Route:

Distance: Time:

NOTES:

Cross-training:

## SATURDAY

Route:

Distance: Time:

NOTES:

Cross-training:

## SUNDAY

Route:

Distance: Time:

NOTES:

Cross-training:

## NOTES

WEEKLY MILEAGE TOTAL:

TOTAL MILEAGE TO DATE:

## INJURY

Snow and ice can make things very dicey. When you do run or walk, don't worry about how fast or slow you're going. Just get into a rhythm that feels easy and comfortable.

## TRAINING

Strides (also called "pick-ups") flood the muscles with blood, recruit your fast-twitch muscle fibers, and help your body transition to running mode. Here's how to do them: After a warmup, gradually accelerate over 60 to 100 meters, then decelerate. After each stride, walk and shake out your legs for 90 seconds. Then stride back in the opposite direction. Strides should not be timed, and the exact distance of each stride is not critical.

## JEREMY OLIVER

Vice president at a community bank
Columbia, Mississippi

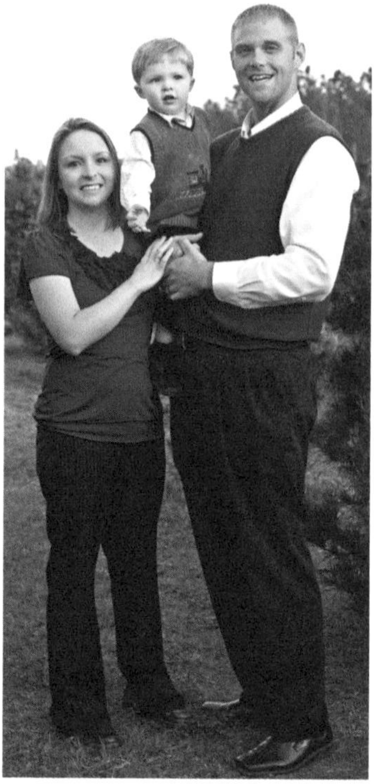

**WHAT GOT ME GOING:** When I found out my wife was pregnant in 2009, I wasn't exercising and I weighed 400 pounds. I wanted to be around for my son, and I knew that I wouldn't be able to if I didn't change something. I had tried exercise programs before, but I never got to a point where it was part of my daily routine. I knew that I had to start exercising, and I had to do it in a way that I could stick with it.

**SECRET OF MY SUCCESS:** Starting small and adding a little bit at a time. When you're 400 pounds, you can't just get out there and run the mile. So I'd go out to a track and run the straightaways and walk the rest of the lap. Each time I'd go out and add a straightaway and eventually got to a point where I could run one time around the track. That was a huge milestone. Now I'm not even getting my heart rate up when I'm running that far.

**HOW RUNNING CHANGED MY LIFE:** It's hard to put into words how much better I feel. I lost nearly 150 pounds. Before, I'd come home from work and want to do absolutely nothing. Now I have energy to help my wife make dinner and clean the house. At work I feel more involved, and I have the confidence to talk to management. I feel like a brand new human being—like I have a second chance in life. I'm a lot happier in my marriage, and a lot of daily problems just don't seem as important anymore.

**I WISH I'D KNOWN:** I didn't realize that there's a science to running, to what kind of shoes to have and clothes to wear. Maybe if I had done more research I wouldn't have had so many false starts and run until I got hurt and couldn't run. Once you start reading, you realize there may be things you're doing on your runs that are hurting you. The more knowledge you have about running and doing it the right way, the better you feel.

# FOR BEGINNERS ONLY

**Q** Is there a minimum amount of running to keep my fitness up? During the winter, between the short days and the snow and ice, I have a hard time finding the time or a safe place to work out. I don't want to lose all the fitness I worked so hard to build.

**A** This is a great question. Even for the most dedicated runner, during certain times of year, like the winter, it's just tough and sometimes impossible to get your regular running workout in. But that doesn't mean you have to give up your exercise goals. Winter is the perfect time to crosstrain and build a foundation of fitness that can make you into a better runner as soon as you can get outside again.

To keep up your running fitness, you want to run a minimum of 10 to 15 miles a week. Try to run 3 miles twice a week with a slightly longer weekend run of 4 to 5 miles. If you have access to a treadmill, or an indoor track, it's perfectly fine to do the miles there. Often runners ask whether miles done indoors "count" or provide the same fitness benefits as outside runs. The answer is: absolutely!

When running just isn't an option, create a flexible exercise schedule that allows you to maintain your fitness and freshen up your routine. You might use the elliptical trainer or the StairMaster as an alternative. Indoor swimming, a rowing ergometer, cycling, or spin classes are also forms of aerobic exercise. You can substitute these options for running, or alternate them with your running days. If you're substituting a cross-training activity for a run, try to work out for the same amount of time at the same level of effort that you'd spend running. You can also take advantage of the winter months to develop more muscular strength, endurance, and flexibility. Weight training sessions, yoga, Pilates, or core strength classes can all help you run more efficiently and stay injury free.

By performing a variety of exercises, you allow your running muscles to recover even while you are still exercising because you are using different muscles in different ways. Do give yourself at least 1 day off each week for complete rest. Your body needs time to recover and adapt to the demands of all these activities. In the long run, this downtime will serve you well by reducing your risk of injury and give you a rested body that is ready to perform.

By maintaining a minimum of 10 to 15 miles a week, adding other aerobic activities and strength training to your routine, you can emerge from winter feeling stronger, more flexible, and ready to run your best.

*Coach and exercise physiologist Susan Paul, author of "For Beginners Only" column,* Runner's World, *is program manager for the Track Shack Foundation. Paul has coached is program director for the Orlando Track Shack Foundation. For more information, visit trackshack.com.*

## NUTRITION

Don't skip meals. Eating three meals each day keeps your metabolism revved, keeps you burning calories, and prevents you from getting ravenous. If you restrict your meals, you'll be more likely to go overboard as soon as anything edible is within arm's reach. Women should aim for 300 to 500 calories per meal. Men should aim for 400 to 600 calories per meal. Both can aim for a 100- to 200-calorie snack.

## MONDAY

Route:

Distance: Time:

NOTES:

Cross-training:

## TUESDAY

Route:

Distance: Time:

NOTES:

Cross-training:

## WEDNESDAY

Route:

Distance: Time:

NOTES:

Cross-training:

## THURSDAY

Route:

Distance: Time:

NOTES:

Cross-training:

## FRIDAY

Route:

Distance: Time:

NOTES:

Cross-training:

"I found hope, love, recovery, and life in running. In so many ways, it changed my life forever."

—**CHRISTINE CASADY,** runner, East Norriton, Pennsylvania, runnersworld.com/christine-casady

## SATURDAY

Route:

Distance: Time:

NOTES:

Cross-training:

## SUNDAY

Route:

Distance: Time:

NOTES:

Cross-training:

## NOTES

WEEKLY MILEAGE TOTAL:

TOTAL MILEAGE TO DATE:

### INJURY

If your shoelace gets untied or you start to chafe early in a workout, take care of it as soon as possible, so it doesn't derail your run. Little issues can lead to big problems if you don't address them.

### TRAINING

Static stretching has been hotly debated in recent years. There is no evidence that it prevents injury or improves performance, experts now say. In fact there's some evidence that it can hurt. Your time before your run is better spent warming up. Or you can do dynamic stretching, which uses controlled leg movements to improve range of motion; loosens up muscles; and increases heart rate, body temperature, and blood flow to help you run more efficiently.

# WEEK 8 WEEK OF ______ TO ______

## NUTRITION

If you're exercising for up to an hour at an easy effort, it's okay to run on an empty stomach. But having a small snack or meal ahead of time may help you feel energized and strong throughout the workout.

"It took me a long time to realize that the runner's high wasn't total crap. I fell off the treadmill once and landed on my face. My legs would cramp up. But every day I was able to go out a little bit longer or feel a little bit better afterward. So I'd go in next day, talk myself down from the fear again. And there was a sense of freedom, even when it was hard, because I could make my legs work like that."

—**JODI EDWARDS,** runner, Lexington Park, Maryland, runnersworld.com/jodi-edwards

## MONDAY

Route:

Distance: Time:

NOTES:

Cross-training:

## TUESDAY

Route:

Distance: Time:

NOTES:

Cross-training:

## WEDNESDAY

Route:

Distance: Time:

NOTES:

Cross-training:

## THURSDAY

Route:

Distance: Time:

NOTES:

Cross-training:

## FRIDAY

Route:

Distance: Time:

NOTES:

Cross-training:

## SATURDAY

Route:

Distance: Time:

NOTES:

Cross-training:

## SUNDAY

Route:

Distance: Time:

NOTES:

Cross-training:

## NOTES

WEEKLY MILEAGE TOTAL:

TOTAL MILEAGE TO DATE:

## INJURY

Orthopedists treat issues affecting the bones, muscles, tendons, and ligaments, which makes them a smart choice if you have an ongoing pain that acts up during or after a run. They are best for running injuries like muscle strains and pulls, joint pains and sprains, and stress fractures. See an orthopedist with a sports medicine specialization who works with athletes to prevent and manage injury. While orthopedists often perform surgery, look for one who is rehab oriented and operates as a last resort.

## TRAINING

Try to think of yourself gliding forward as you run. When you're just starting out, it's natural to tend to bounce up and down, which wastes a lot of energy and slows you down. Run like you've got a really low ceiling overhead that you don't want to hit.

## NUTRITION

About half of each meal should be carbs, including whole grains, fruits, and vegetables. Not only are fruits and veggies low in calories, high in fiber, and filling, but a wide variety of produce will provide nutrients and minerals that help stave off diseases like cancer and keep your bones, muscles, metabolism, heart, and lungs in top form.

"Your greatest runs are rarely measured by racing success. They are moments in time when running allows you to see how wonderful your life is."

—KARA GOUCHER, Olympic marathoner

### MONDAY

Route:

Distance: Time:

NOTES:

Cross-training:

### TUESDAY

Route:

Distance: Time:

NOTES:

Cross-training:

### WEDNESDAY

Route:

Distance: Time:

NOTES:

Cross-training:

### THURSDAY

Route:

Distance: Time:

NOTES:

Cross-training:

### FRIDAY

Route:

Distance: Time:

NOTES:

Cross-training:

## SATURDAY

Route:

Distance: Time:

NOTES:

Cross-training:

## SUNDAY

Route:

Distance: Time:

NOTES:

Cross-training:

## NOTES

## WEEKLY MILEAGE TOTAL:

## TOTAL MILEAGE TO DATE:

### INJURY

When you're running, assume that a driver can't see you. Always run or walk facing traffic so you can see, and react to, oncoming cars. If traffic gets heavy, or the road narrows, be prepared to move onto the sidewalk or shoulder of the road. Wear high-visibility, brightly colored clothing. When out near or after sunset, reflective materials are a must. And use a headlamp so you can see where you're going, and drivers can see you.

### TRAINING

Fartlek, or speed play in Swedish, is a workout in which you alternate between faster and slower intervals of running, making each interval as long (or short) as you want.

## NUTRITION

What's the perfect preworkout meal? Familiar foods that are easy on your system, low in fat and fiber, and high in carbs will boost your energy without upsetting your stomach. Try graham crackers and honey, fig cookies, or a banana with 1 tablespoon of peanut, almond, or cashew butter.

## MONDAY

Route:

Distance: Time:

NOTES:

Cross-training:

## TUESDAY

Route:

Distance: Time:

NOTES:

Cross-training:

## WEDNESDAY

Route:

Distance: Time:

NOTES:

Cross-training:

## THURSDAY

Route:

Distance: Time:

NOTES:

Cross-training:

## FRIDAY

Route:

Distance: Time:

NOTES:

Cross-training:

"Our greatest glory is not in never falling, but in rising every time we fall."

—CONFUCIUS

## SATURDAY

Route:

Distance: Time:

NOTES:

Cross-training:

## SUNDAY

Route:

Distance: Time:

NOTES:

Cross-training:

## NOTES

WEEKLY MILEAGE TOTAL:

TOTAL MILEAGE TO DATE:

## INJURY

The one thing that's absolutely, positively known about running injuries is that old injuries lead to future injuries, says Amby Burfoot, *Runner's World* editor at large and winner of the 1968 Boston Marathon. The key, then, is to avoid injury the first time around. Today you might have a tender spot on your shin. Keep running, and it could become a full-fledged injury that leads to chronic problems or to other counterbalance injuries. You could spend a lifetime regretting the days when you continued running; you'll never regret the 3 to 7 days of rest.

## TRAINING

If you're walking, your cadence should feel quick. You should be able to hold a conversation. If you can sing, you're likely going too slow. If you are huffing and puffing, you're going too fast.

## NUTRITION

Overindulging your sweet tooth can lead to weight gain and health problems like type 2 diabetes and high blood pressure. Look for products with the fewest grams of sugar, and aim for less than 2.5 grams of sugar per 100 calories. The World Health Organization recommends keeping sugar intake to no more than 10 percent of daily calories. For many folks that's a limit of 50 grams of sugar per day. Aim much lower if you're trying to shed pounds. Your best source of sugar is fresh fruit, which provides vitamins and minerals along with fiber.

"Find your own play, your own compulsion, and you will become the person you are meant to be."

—DR. GEORGE SHEEHAN, author and former columnist for *Runner's World*

### MONDAY

Route:

Distance: Time:

NOTES:

Cross-training:

### TUESDAY

Route:

Distance: Time:

NOTES:

Cross-training:

### WEDNESDAY

Route:

Distance: Time:

NOTES:

Cross-training:

### THURSDAY

Route:

Distance: Time:

NOTES:

Cross-training:

### FRIDAY

Route:

Distance: Time:

NOTES:

Cross-training:

## SATURDAY

Route:

Distance: Time:

NOTES:

Cross-training:

## SUNDAY

Route:

Distance: Time:

NOTES:

Cross-training:

## NOTES

WEEKLY MILEAGE TOTAL:

TOTAL MILEAGE TO DATE:

### INJURY

When in doubt, rest and have your pain checked out. It's better to spend a little time and money seeing the doctor than to be sidelined for months by an injury that you could have prevented or minimized.

### TRAINING

The softer surface that trails offer can be great if you've struggled with overuse injuries like runner's knee, iliotibial-band syndrome (ITBS), or shin splints. Just be wary of "technical" trails with lots of roots, rocks, and uneven ground that cause your feet to land at an angle. Look for trails that are identified as dirt, asphalt, or even paved Rails-to-Trails routes.

## NUTRITION

Even as you get fitter, you may not see results on the scale right away. Keep in mind: Muscle weighs more than fat, and hydration, hormones, time of day, and other factors can all have an impact on the numbers on the scale. Don't measure success with the scale alone. Are your pants getting looser? Are you getting more compliments? Do you have more energy? What about your blood pressure, cholesterol, and other markers of chronic disease? All these are even more important measures of fitness success.

"Mind is everything; muscles, mere pieces of rubber. All that I am, I am because of my mind."

—**PAAVO NURMI**, 12-time Olympic gold medalist

### MONDAY

Route:

Distance: Time:

NOTES:

Cross-training:

### TUESDAY

Route:

Distance: Time:

NOTES:

Cross-training:

### WEDNESDAY

Route:

Distance: Time:

NOTES:

Cross-training:

### THURSDAY

Route:

Distance: Time:

NOTES:

Cross-training:

### FRIDAY

Route:

Distance: Time:

NOTES:

Cross-training:

## SATURDAY

Route:

Distance: Time:

NOTES:

Cross-training:

## SUNDAY

Route:

Distance: Time:

NOTES:

Cross-training:

## NOTES

WEEKLY MILEAGE TOTAL:

TOTAL MILEAGE TO DATE:

## INJURY

While the cushioned surface of a treadmill helps prevent injuries, some people report aches and pains after putting in extra time on the 'mill. Be sure to run at a pace you can comfortably sustain. As you tire, lower your speed or the incline. If you can't keep up with the treadmill without grabbing the handrails, you're going too fast. Holding on to the handrails can throw off your stride and create a twisting motion, which can lead to injuries.

## TRAINING

If you've done 100 percent of your workouts on a treadmill, gradually integrate outdoor running into your routine. Too quick a transition can lead to injury. On your first outside run, start with 10 minutes, and add 5 minutes the next week. Continue to build gradually.

## DARLENE ANITA SCOTT

University instructor and writer
Richmond, Virginia

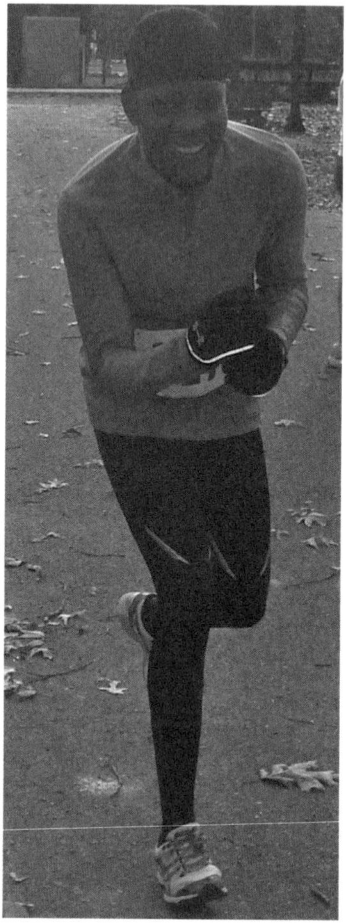

**WHAT GOT ME GOING:** I stopped dating this guy I liked and was determined that the next time he saw me he would regret it. (I think my plan worked!) That also prompted me to start thinking more about how much I'd been stifling myself. I began doing a bunch of stuff I had wanted to do, from running to painting to skydiving to swim lessons.

**SECRET OF MY SUCCESS:** I felt like an outsider in fitness communities. I had been a sedentary kid and was known in my family as the clumsy and awkward one. I'm still getting over the internalization of that, but I found outfits that made me feel like I "looked the part" and found that I internalized that until it became who I was or at least someone I could be.

**HOW RUNNING CHANGED MY LIFE:** I've met people who will be my friends for life and I've found confidence I did not realize I lacked. Both of these helped me in other parts of my life.

**I WISH I'D KNOWN:** Don't try to sprint on your first day! I think we get it into our heads that we need to go fast—like we're running the races we ran as kids. Then we get discouraged about our ability (or what we perceive as a lack of it). Someone told me to go at a comfortable pace for as long as I could. I did and surprised myself by how much I could do—which motivated me to see what else I could do. You won't come back if your first experience sucks.

# FOR BEGINNERS ONLY

**Q** What are the right walking and running speeds?

**A** The appropriate or ideal speed is relative to each individual and his or her current fitness level. Rather than go by speed alone, it might be a better bet to monitor your heart rate, your breathing rate, and/or your Rate of Perceived Exertion (RPE) to measure your effort. If you're using a heart rate monitor, your physician may also give you some recommendations for the exercise heart rate range to maintain while you're exercising; if so, adjust your treadmill speed and incline to achieve that range.

A general heart rate guideline is the range of 60 to 80 percent of your maximum heart rate during most of your workouts. If you are not accustomed to taking your heart rate, you can also gauge exercise intensity by your breathing rate and how you feel. Just like your heart rate, your breathing rate will increase with exercise, but you should still be able to speak while walking or running. If you cannot speak, slow it down; on the other hand, if you can sing, then pick up the pace! Another easy way to monitor exercise intensity is by your RPE. Simply put, if the exercise feels easy, it is easy; if it feels hard, it is hard. Adjust your pace, up or down, according to how you feel. You want a pace that makes you sweat, increases heart rate, increases breathing rate, and burns calories; but also a pace that you can maintain for the duration of the exercise session. Duration is very important, especially when beginning a training plan; better to do 20 or 30 minutes at a slower pace than to last only 10 minutes at a faster pace. Also, expect to adjust your pace periodically.

For most people 2 to 4 mph will be a walking speed; 4 to 5 mph will be a very fast walk or jog; and anything over 5 mph will be jogging or running.

As your fitness level improves, you will need to walk or run faster and longer to continue building your aerobic and muscular strength and endurance. If you are more comfortable at a walking pace but wish to increase the intensity of the exercise, you can add more incline to achieve the intensity level or heart rate range you desire. Play with both variables of speed and incline to find what works best for you.

Since your running focuses on improving your cardio-respiratory system, on your "off" days try working on your muscular strength, endurance, and flexibility with weight training, core classes, yoga, or Pilates. These are also very important fitness components too, and they will help make you a better walker or runner and stay injury free.

*Coach and exercise physiologist Susan Paul, author of "For Beginners Only" column,* Runner's World, *is program manager for the Track Shack Foundation. Paul has coached is program director for the Orlando Track Shack Foundation. For more information, visit trackshack.com.*

## NUTRITION

The "calories burned" readouts on exercise machines are often not accurate. That's because many treadmills estimate total calories burned rather than the net number—for example, calories burned solely through exercise, above and beyond what we would have used anyway. Plus, most machines don't account for body-fat percentage, gender, age, resting heart rate, or whether you're holding on to the rails.

"I run to get rid of stress. I run to lose weight. I run when I'm mad, and when I'm sad. All the things that used to make me light up a cigarette now make me put my running shoes on."

—**KELLY CASSIDY**, runner, Milford, Michigan, runnersworld.com/kelly-cassidy

### MONDAY

Route:

Distance: Time:

NOTES:

Cross-training:

### TUESDAY

Route:

Distance: Time:

NOTES:

Cross-training:

### WEDNESDAY

Route:

Distance: Time:

NOTES:

Cross-training:

### THURSDAY

Route:

Distance: Time:

NOTES:

Cross-training:

### FRIDAY

Route:

Distance: Time:

NOTES:

Cross-training:

## SATURDAY

Route:

Distance: Time:

NOTES:

Cross-training:

## SUNDAY

Route:

Distance: Time:

NOTES:

Cross-training:

## NOTES

WEEKLY MILEAGE TOTAL:

TOTAL MILEAGE TO DATE:

## INJURY

Lots of downhill running and too-small shoes can cause black toenails, because both situations cause your toes to slam into the front of your shoe. They typically heal on their own within a few weeks.

## TRAINING

Don't worry about your pace or miles covered when you're just starting out. The first step is to focus on building overall fitness—and to make exercise a habit. The main health benefits, from lower risk of cardiovascular disease, diabetes, and hypertension, result from the time you consistently spend elevating your heart rate.

WEEK 14 WEEK OF ______ TO ______

## NUTRITION

After a tough workout, you may not be hungry right away. But it's best to have small snack as soon as you can stomach it. That will prevent you from getting famished and going overboard later. Studies have shown that it's easy for runners to eat back their calories after tough workouts.

"Be positive, ignore the critic, follow your heart, invest in your passions, believe in your dreams, and get busy making them reality."

—**JOSH COX,** U.S. 50-K record holder

### MONDAY

Route:

Distance: Time:

NOTES:

Cross-training:

### TUESDAY

Route:

Distance: Time:

NOTES:

Cross-training:

### WEDNESDAY

Route:

Distance: Time:

NOTES:

Cross-training:

### THURSDAY

Route:

Distance: Time:

NOTES:

Cross-training:

### FRIDAY

Route:

Distance: Time:

NOTES:

Cross-training:

## SATURDAY
Route:

Distance: Time:

NOTES:

Cross-training:

## SUNDAY
Route:

Distance: Time:

NOTES:

Cross-training:

## NOTES

WEEKLY MILEAGE TOTAL:

TOTAL MILEAGE TO DATE:

## INJURY
Bloody nipples are often caused by chafing, friction caused by the rubbing of the nipples against the shirt while running. They're more common in men and during cold weather, and they can be remedied by covering your nipples with adhesive bandages or nipple guards, which are sold in many specialty running stores.

## TRAINING
It's important to take walk breaks before you feel like you need them. This will help fend off fatigue and prevent you from doing too much too soon. By taking walk breaks at the regular intervals that are scheduled for the day, you can ensure that you'll finish each workout feeling strong.

WEEK 15 WEEK OF ____ TO ____

## NUTRITION

For an easy workout of 1 hour or less, going without food or drink probably won't do you any harm. (Just make sure you're staying hydrated.) But for any event that's longer or more intense, preworkout fuel is critical. Go out on empty and you'll fatigue sooner, plus you'll have a much tougher time meeting your goals.

"Do not give up when it gets tough. It gets better. And it will be the best feeling in the world to say you are a runner."

—**JOHN MCNASBY,** runner, Philadelphia, runnersworld.com/john-mcnasby

## MONDAY

Route:

Distance: Time:

NOTES:

Cross-training:

## TUESDAY

Route:

Distance: Time:

NOTES:

Cross-training:

## WEDNESDAY

Route:

Distance: Time:

NOTES:

Cross-training:

## THURSDAY

Route:

Distance: Time:

NOTES:

Cross-training:

## FRIDAY

Route:

Distance: Time:

NOTES:

Cross-training:

## SATURDAY
Route:

Distance: Time:

NOTES:

Cross-training:

## SUNDAY
Route:

Distance: Time:

NOTES:

Cross-training:

## NOTES

WEEKLY MILEAGE TOTAL:

TOTAL MILEAGE TO DATE:

## INJURY
When it's hot and humid outside, check the heat index. It's a combined measurement of temperature and humidity that shows how hot it feels outside. When humidity is high, it interferes with the body's ability to sweat—and cool itself—so the body retains more heat and it's riskier to be outside. High humidity also increases the risk for heat cramps, heat exhaustion, and heatstroke.

## TRAINING
Once you hit a pace that feels comfortable, tune in to how your body feels. How hard are you breathing? How quickly are your legs turning over? How do your leg muscles feel? Getting a sense of how your comfortable pace feels will help you dial into it on every run.

WEEK 16 WEEK OF TO

## NUTRITION

The bigger the meal the more time you'll need to digest. Each person is different, but for most people it's best to eat at least 30 minutes before heading out to avoid GI distress when you're on the road. Within 20 minutes of finishing your workout, have a protein-rich snack to repair muscle tissue and carbohydrates to restock your spent energy stores. This will kick-start the recovery process so that you can bounce back quickly for your next workout.

"Winning doesn't always mean getting first place; it means getting the best out of yourself."

—**MEB KEFLEZIGHI,** Olympic marathoner

## MONDAY

**Route:**

**Distance:** **Time:**

**NOTES:**

**Cross-training:**

## TUESDAY

**Route:**

**Distance:** **Time:**

**NOTES:**

**Cross-training:**

## WEDNESDAY

**Route:**

**Distance:** **Time:**

**NOTES:**

**Cross-training:**

## THURSDAY

**Route:**

**Distance:** **Time:**

**NOTES:**

**Cross-training:**

## FRIDAY

**Route:**

**Distance:** **Time:**

**NOTES:**

**Cross-training:**

## SATURDAY

**Route:**

**Distance:** **Time:**

**NOTES:**

**Cross-training:**

## SUNDAY

**Route:**

**Distance:** **Time:**

**NOTES:**

**Cross-training:**

## NOTES

## WEEKLY MILEAGE TOTAL:

## TOTAL MILEAGE TO DATE:

## INJURY

The term RICE refers to Rest, Ice, Compression, and Elevation. These measures can relieve pain, reduce swelling, and protect damaged tissues, all of which speed healing. They're most effective when done immediately following an injury. RICE is the standard prescription for many aches and pains, such as strained hamstrings and twisted ankles.

## TRAINING

When you first start out, it's common to clench up muscles that aren't involved in running. And that can sap the strength you need for a good workout. So when the going gets tough, do a body scan: Unknit your brow, unclench your jaw, keep your hands relaxed (imagine holding a piece of paper between your thumb and pointer finger), and don't forget to breathe. You'll be amazed at how much easier the workout feels!

## NUTRITION

A flood of low-fat and fat-free products have entered the market. But unsaturated fats like the ones you can get from olive oil, avocados, canola oil, nuts, seeds, and almonds actually help boost your heart health. They also leave you feeling fuller for longer. Stay away from saturated fat and trans fat; they raise your "bad" cholesterol levels and decrease your "good" cholesterol levels, and that can raise your risk for heart disease. You still want to keep fats in moderation.

"Running made me feel like a bird let out of a cage. I loved it that much."

—PRISCILLA WELCH, 1987 New York City Marathon winner

## MONDAY

Route:

Distance: Time:

NOTES:

Cross-training:

## TUESDAY

Route:

Distance: Time:

NOTES:

Cross-training:

## WEDNESDAY

Route:

Distance: Time:

NOTES:

Cross-training:

## THURSDAY

Route:

Distance: Time:

NOTES:

Cross-training:

## FRIDAY

Route:

Distance: Time:

NOTES:

Cross-training:

## SATURDAY

Route:

Distance: Time:

NOTES:

Cross-training:

## SUNDAY

Route:

Distance: Time:

NOTES:

Cross-training:

## NOTES

WEEKLY MILEAGE TOTAL:

TOTAL MILEAGE TO DATE:

## INJURY

A side stitch is a sharp pain usually felt just below the rib cage. It's thought to be caused by a cramp in the diaphragm, gas in the intestines, or food in the stomach. To get rid of a side stitch, notice which foot is striking the ground when you inhale and exhale, then switch the pattern. So if you were leading with your right foot, inhale when your left foot steps. If that doesn't help, stop running and reach both arms above your head. Bend at your waist, leaning to the side opposite the stitch until the pain subsides.

## TRAINING

Winter is not the time to be rigid about when, where, and how far you go. If you're a morning exerciser, switch to midday workouts when the air is the warmest. If you run on trails, you may need to stick to well-lit roads or the treadmill.

## NUTRITION

When you're trying to lose weight, you don't have to completely opt out of eating out. Many restaurants offer calorie and nutrition information for their meals, online or by request. If you know you're going to be heading out to eat, research the menu ahead of time so you know what the healthy options are and can plan what to order. Don't hesitate to ask about how a dish is prepared, what ingredients are included, or request that sauces and dressings be served on the side. Order first, so you're not swayed by someone else's less healthy order if it sounds tempting.

"On every run, I discover the strength that I did not know I had."

—**CARRIE PARKER,** runner, Deer Island, New Brunswick, Canada, runnersworld.com/carrie-parker

### MONDAY

Route:

Distance: Time:

NOTES:

Cross-training:

### TUESDAY

Route:

Distance: Time:

NOTES:

Cross-training:

### WEDNESDAY

Route:

Distance: Time:

NOTES:

Cross-training:

### THURSDAY

Route:

Distance: Time:

NOTES:

Cross-training:

### FRIDAY

Route:

Distance: Time:

NOTES:

Cross-training:

## SATURDAY

Route:

Distance: Time:

NOTES:

Cross-training:

## SUNDAY

Route:

Distance: Time:

NOTES:

Cross-training:

## NOTES

WEEKLY MILEAGE TOTAL:

TOTAL MILEAGE TO DATE:

## INJURY

Stride rate is the number of times your feet hit the ground during a minute of running. This measurement is often used to assess running efficiency. Having a high stride rate—say 170 steps per minute or more—can reduce injuries and help you get faster. Typically the number used refers to the total number of times either foot hits the ground. So for a person with a stride rate of 170, the right foot and the left foot would each have hit the ground 85 times.

## TRAINING

Start each workout slow. If you go out too fast, you run the risk of pulling a muscle, tweaking a tendon, bone, or joint, or getting into a pace that you can't sustain. The result? You end up slowing down and burning out before you're done with your workout. The worst part is that you're likely to end your run feeling exhausted and discouraged and dreading your next workout.

## RUFFIN RHODES

Architect
Oviedo, Florida

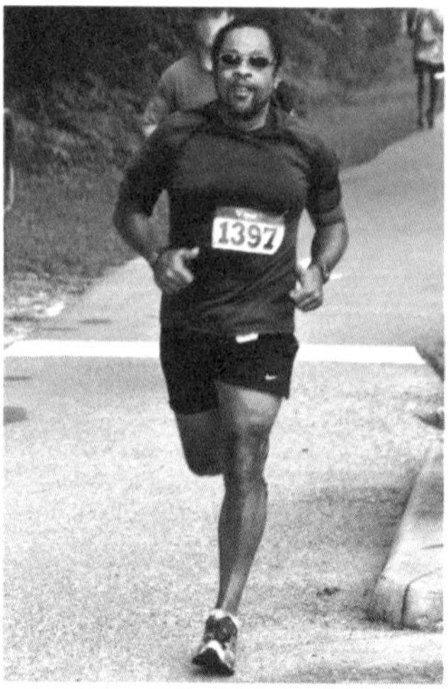

**WHAT GOT ME GOING:** In January of 2008, at the age of 49, I was 5'6", weighed 250 pounds, and was on high blood pressure medication. Diabetes is prevalent in my family history, and my father suffered from it. I watched him inject insulin several times daily, take medication for hypertension and congestive heart failure. He was also obese and as an indirect result of obesity, he finally succumbed to a heart attack several years later. Having watched his struggles with obesity and diabetes, I knew diabetes would soon be knocking on my door. I have a wife and two children, and I realized I needed to get serious about my health.

**SECRET OF MY SUCCESS:** I started walking, stopped eating fast food, and began counting my calorie intake. A year later, I joined a gym and started working out on an elliptical trainer, lifting weights, and eventually running on the treadmill. I began getting up at 4 a.m. to challenge my commitment. Previously at work, I ate on the run, grabbing fast foods and going out to restaurants. Now I bring my lunches to work and refuse lunch meetings, and my wife and I rarely go out to eat but elect to stay home and cook a healthy meal and then go to a movie. I'm a fanatic about weighing my food. I have a scale at home and at the office.

**HOW RUNNING CHANGED MY LIFE:** I now run up to 25 miles a week and lift weights twice a week. I'm down to 176 pounds. Running has made me a much more disciplined and confident professional. I have more energy to spend time with my children, and it's benefited my marriage. Running, for me, is like a cheap therapy session. As an architect and partner in my own company, I'm often stressed. Many times I've resolved work problems or design solutions while out on my runs. It's the solitude that allows me to think a bit more clearly and de-stress.

**I WISH I'D KNOWN:** Invest in good running shoes. When I first tried running, I tried running on some cheap cross-trainers and was constantly battling knee pain. I was about to give up until a friend recommended I get sized for a proper pair of running shoes. It was the best $140 I ever spent, and it made all the difference in the world.

# FOR BEGINNERS ONLY

**Q** How do I transition from walking to running?

**A** Walking has given you a great base of conditioning. Keep your walking going and then to begin running, try adding some very small increments of run time interspersed throughout your walking routine. For example, warmup first by walking for several minutes. Then run at an easy pace for just 30 seconds; then walk for 2 to 3 minutes. Add another short run interval of 30 seconds after you feel recovered. Repeat this run/walk sequence throughout your exercise session. Play with the time intervals for both the run and the walk portions based on how you feel; however, starting with very short run intervals and longer walk intervals is the way to begin. Gradually increase the length of the run intervals by small increments of time over a period of several months. Most likely, during this process you will find a run/walk interval you feel comfortable with and enjoy using.

Also, watch your running pace. Often when new runners find they cannot maintain a run, it's because they are running too fast. If you find you cannot maintain your run pace, slow down, return to walking, and recover. Once recovered, try running again at a slower pace. It's important to note that many runners use a run/walk interval as their training method, so it's not just for beginners. There is no hard and fast rule that states you must run continuously to be a runner.

Be patient with your progress. Our bodies take time to adapt to the demands of exercise, much longer than we realize. As a general rule of thumb, it takes the body about 6 weeks to adapt to the training stimulus. And the older we are, the longer the adaptation process takes. Your dedication and consistency are impressive.

Monitoring your resting heart rate (RHR) is a good way to track your fitness gains. Take your resting pulse each morning, before getting out of bed, for 1 minute and record it. As your fitness level improves, your resting pulse declines. After several heart rate readings, you will have your current baseline. When you see your RHR drop, you will know your body is adapting to the training and becoming fitter. When you see a rise in your resting heart rate of 10 beats or more, it's a red flag. A higher-than-normal RHR can indicate a variety of problems, whether it's an oncoming illness, lack of recovery, not getting enough sleep, overtraining, stress, or dehydration. Whatever the cause, it lets you know you should back off from the day's workout. Sleep in, take the workout at an easier pace, or cut a long run short. When your RHR returns to normal, you will know your body is ready for a workout.

*Coach and exercise physiologist Susan Paul, author of "For Beginners Only" column,* Runner's World, *is program manager for the Track Shack Foundation. Paul has coached is program director for the Orlando Track Shack Foundation. For more information, visit trackshack.com.*

## NUTRITION

Try to stick with drinking water most of the time, but low-fat milk, recovery drinks, sports drinks, and even some 100% fruit juices can offer some health benefits. Just avoid fancy drinks, some of which can pack a meal's worth of calories into a single glass. They add nothing to your diet but unwanted calories that quickly turn into unwanted pounds.

"As a breed, runners are a pretty gutsy bunch. We constantly push ourselves to discover limitations, then push past them. We want to know how fast we can go, how much pain we can endure, and how far our bodies can carry us before collapsing in exhaustion."

—**BART YASSO,** *Runner's World* chief running officer

### MONDAY

**Route:**

**Distance:** **Time:**

**NOTES:**

**Cross-training:**

### TUESDAY

**Route:**

**Distance:** **Time:**

**NOTES:**

**Cross-training:**

### WEDNESDAY

**Route:**

**Distance:** **Time:**

**NOTES:**

**Cross-training:**

### THURSDAY

**Route:**

**Distance:** **Time:**

**NOTES:**

**Cross-training:**

### FRIDAY

**Route:**

**Distance:** **Time:**

**NOTES:**

**Cross-training:**

## SATURDAY

Route:

Distance: Time:

NOTES:

Cross-training:

## SUNDAY

Route:

Distance: Time:

NOTES:

Cross-training:

## NOTES

WEEKLY MILEAGE TOTAL:

TOTAL MILEAGE TO DATE:

### INJURY

Stay safe on the road. Tell somebody or leave a note at home about where you plan to go and how long you plan to be out. That way your loved ones will know to come look for you if needed. Identify yourself. Run with proper ID and carry a cell phone with emergency contacts taped to its back.

### TRAINING

Your running pace may vary greatly from day to day, depending on the weather, your fatigue level, and many other factors. While it's good to have a general idea of how fast you're running, it's best not to focus too much on hitting certain paces all the time. Doing so usually leads to working too hard and can drain much of the enjoyment from your running. As you gain fitness, you'll naturally speed up.

WEEK OF ______ TO ______

## NUTRITION

Eat your spinach! It delivers tons of nutrients you need with few calories. With less than 10 calories per cup, spinach is packed with iron, potassium, and antioxidant vitamins like A, C, and K.

### MONDAY

Route:

Distance: Time:

NOTES:

Cross-training:

### TUESDAY

Route:

Distance: Time:

NOTES:

Cross-training:

### WEDNESDAY

Route:

Distance: Time:

NOTES:

Cross-training:

### THURSDAY

Route:

Distance: Time:

NOTES:

Cross-training:

### FRIDAY

Route:

Distance: Time:

NOTES:

Cross-training:

"Truly, I love running. It's who I am. It's a part of me. Even if I can only run for 10 minutes, I feel whole and happy. And if everything else is falling to pieces, I go for a run, and I feel like things are going to be okay."

—JOHANNA OLSON, Olympic marathon trials runner who died of brain cancer at the age of 33

## SATURDAY

Route:

Distance: Time:

NOTES:

Cross-training:

## SUNDAY

Route:

Distance: Time:

NOTES:

Cross-training:

## NOTES

WEEKLY MILEAGE TOTAL:

TOTAL MILEAGE TO DATE:

## INJURY

When you first start out, the trick is to be consistent enough that you're building strength and endurance, yet slow enough that you don't get hurt. In order to do that, you're going to need to do all of your training at an easy pace. Get into a rhythm that feels like you could maintain it forever. It should feel comfortable and conversational. Develop endurance first; speed will come later.

## TRAINING

Quality workouts typically refer to any workouts that are faster or longer than daily runs. Within the context of race training, the term usually refers to workouts such as long runs, speed sessions, and tempo runs, which all require a day or two of rest.

# WEEK 21 WEEK OF TO

## NUTRITION

If you're cutting calories or carbs, you may be tempted to eliminate whole grains from your diet. But these are important sources of the energizing vitamins and minerals you need for your workouts. About half of your daily calories should come from carbs that include vegetables, fruits, and whole grains.

"Running has helped me control my disease. I want to show people that you can have a better life through exercise."

—**DOUG MASIUK,** the first type-1 diabetic to run across the country

## MONDAY

Route:

Distance: Time:

NOTES:

Cross-training:

## TUESDAY

Route:

Distance: Time:

NOTES:

Cross-training:

## WEDNESDAY

Route:

Distance: Time:

NOTES:

Cross-training:

## THURSDAY

Route:

Distance: Time:

NOTES:

Cross-training:

## FRIDAY

Route:

Distance: Time:

NOTES:

Cross-training:

## SATURDAY

**Route:**

**Distance:** **Time:**

**NOTES:**

**Cross-training:**

## SUNDAY

**Route:**

**Distance:** **Time:**

**NOTES:**

**Cross-training:**

## NOTES

## WEEKLY MILEAGE TOTAL:

## TOTAL MILEAGE TO DATE:

### INJURY

Overstriding—extending your foot and leg far out in front of your knee—is a common cause of injury. Be sure to keep your steps short and quick as you're doing the strides. Keep your feet and legs underneath your torso.

### TRAINING

The run/walk method popularized by Olympian Jeff Galloway, columnist and author of *Runner's World*'s monthly "Starting Line" column, is a great way to start working out. Walk breaks allow a runner to feel strong to the end and recover fast, while providing the same stamina and conditioning as a continuous run. By shifting back and forth between walking and running, you work a variety of different muscle groups, which helps fend off fatigue.

WEEK OF ____ TO ____

## NUTRITION

Whole grain foods include the bran, germ, and endosperm—which contain the nutritious B vitamins, iron, magnesium, and fiber you need to build strength. When whole grains are refined into foods like white bread, the nutrients are lost, and so is the fiber. Fiber helps lower cholesterol, reduce blood pressure, and decrease the risk of diabetes and heart disease. Fiber also helps the keep the digestive system functioning and keeps you feeling fuller for longer.

"You don't love running when you first start because it hurts. Your legs hurt, your lungs hurt. But once you make the decision and start to move forward, you become a different person. It's not about having to hit your goal weight to start feeling good again."

—**BEN DAVIS**, founder of bendoeslife.com

### MONDAY

Route:

Distance: Time:

NOTES:

Cross-training:

### TUESDAY

Route:

Distance: Time:

NOTES:

Cross-training:

### WEDNESDAY

Route:

Distance: Time:

NOTES:

Cross-training:

### THURSDAY

Route:

Distance: Time:

NOTES:

Cross-training:

### FRIDAY

Route:

Distance: Time:

NOTES:

Cross-training:

## SATURDAY

Route:

Distance: Time:

NOTES:

Cross-training:

## SUNDAY

Route:

Distance: Time:

NOTES:

Cross-training:

## NOTES

WEEKLY MILEAGE TOTAL:

TOTAL MILEAGE TO DATE:

### INJURY

When temperatures climb, head out early or late. Even in the worst heat wave, it is significantly cooler before dawn. Get your run done then, and you'll feel good about it all day. Can't fit it in? Wait until evening, when the sun's rays aren't as strong—just don't do it so late that you can't get to sleep.

### TRAINING

Speedwork, also called intervals or repeats, refers to any workout run at a faster-than-normal pace. Speedwork is often done at a track, but can also be done on a treadmill or a flat stretch of road. You can do speedwork to boost cardiovascular and muscular fitness.

WEEK 23 WEEK OF ______ TO ______

## NUTRITION

If you're going to be on the road for 75 minutes or longer, refuel on the run to stay energized. A variety of energy gels and chews are on the market, or you can use candy or real food. Aim for 30 to 60 grams of carbs per hour while you're on the road. Even if you're not hungry or tired, to prevent bonking, start fueling 20 to 30 minutes into the run and keep refueling at regular intervals. Try lots of different brands and flavors to figure out what flavor and blend gives you a boost without leaving you with an upset stomach.

"I always feel better after running than I did before I started, and I hang on to that. My best mood is only a few miles away!"

—**ANDREA "ANDI" BALL,** runner, Elkridge Park, Maryland, runnersworld.com/andi-ball

### MONDAY

Route:

Distance: Time:

NOTES:

Cross-training:

### TUESDAY

Route:

Distance: Time:

NOTES:

Cross-training:

### WEDNESDAY

Route:

Distance: Time:

NOTES:

Cross-training:

### THURSDAY

Route:

Distance: Time:

NOTES:

Cross-training:

### FRIDAY

Route:

Distance: Time:

NOTES:

Cross-training:

## SATURDAY

Route:

Distance: Time:

NOTES:

Cross-training:

## SUNDAY

Route:

Distance: Time:

NOTES:

Cross-training:

## NOTES

WEEKLY MILEAGE TOTAL:

TOTAL MILEAGE TO DATE:

### INJURY

When it's hot outside, try to work out in the grass and the shade. It's always hotter in cities than in surrounding areas because asphalt and concrete retain heat. If you must run in an urban or even a suburban area, look for shade and try to go in the early morning or late evening.

### TRAINING

Are you running too fast or too slow? Do the talk test. This is a way to see if you're running at a comfortable effort level. During most of your runs, you should be able to carry on a conversation. If you can't say more than a few words at a time, you're probably running too hard. Back off to where you can say a sentence at a time.

## NUTRITION

Certainly it's important to stay hydrated during exercise. But for the average workout of 60 minutes or less, you typically won't need anything more than water. If you're going longer than an hour, or it's hot and humid outside, then you may need the carbohydrates and electrolytes that sports drinks provide.

"I think when you run by someone and there's a thumbs-up or encouragement, that's something that I really love. It's a brotherhood, a support, and an appreciation for the effort we're all making."

—**GENE BAUR,** cofounder and president of Farm Sanctuary

### MONDAY

Route:

Distance: Time:

NOTES:

Cross-training:

### TUESDAY

Route:

Distance: Time:

NOTES:

Cross-training:

### WEDNESDAY

Route:

Distance: Time:

NOTES:

Cross-training:

### THURSDAY

Route:

Distance: Time:

NOTES:

Cross-training:

### FRIDAY

Route:

Distance: Time:

NOTES:

Cross-training:

## SATURDAY

Route:

Distance: Time:

NOTES:

Cross-training:

## SUNDAY

Route:

Distance: Time:

NOTES:

Cross-training:

## NOTES

WEEKLY MILEAGE TOTAL:

TOTAL MILEAGE TO DATE:

## INJURY

Blisters are caused by friction, excessive moisture (sweaty feet, wet weather), or shoes that are too small, too big, or tied too tight. Putting Vaseline, sports lube, and bandages over blister-prone spots may also help. Ignore blisters the size of a pencil eraser, since they're usually not painful. But pop the big ones. With a sterile needle, prick the side of the blister and drain it. Don't remove the top of the blister; instead, cover it with an antibiotic ointment and moleskin or a bandage.

## TRAINING

Once a week you may want to substitute one workout with a pool-running session of the same duration. If you're new to pool running, use a flotation device and simply move your legs as if you were running on land, with a slightly exaggerated forward lean and vigorous arm pump.

## CHRISTIN ACCOMANDO

Corporate communications
Chicago, Illinois

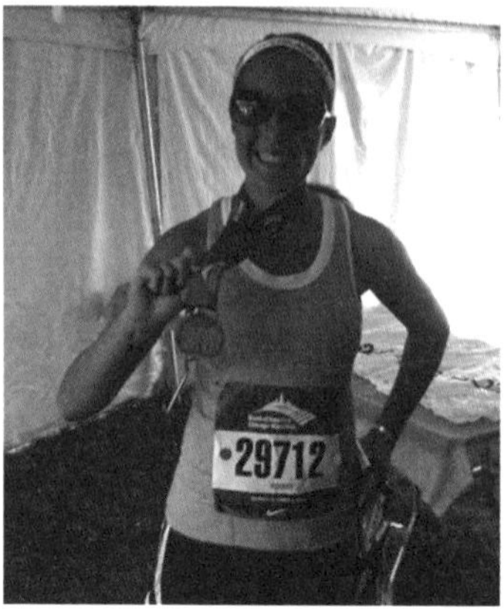


**WHAT GOT ME GOING:** In 2011, I was feeling down, trying to figure out what I wanted to do with my life. A cousin encouraged me to run an 8-K race with him, the Shamrock Shuffle in Chicago. So I took on the challenge and trained for my first nearly 5-mile run. (The most I had run before was a 5-K.) After that race, I fell in love with running and the euphoria of crossing the finish line. Staying in shape has always been a passion of mine because I have cystic fibrosis (CF). But before I started running, my workouts consisted of a few situps and pushups and maybe a 2-mile jog. Ironically, although CF affects my lungs, I feel better when I live an active lifestyle. Nothing has made me feel better than running!

**SECRET OF MY SUCCESS:** Running, especially training for a long-distance race, is very time consuming. It takes commitment and a true passion for the sport. You really have to want it and be willing to make it a priority. I was able to commit by joining a running group. We held each other accountable, encouraged each other, and kicked each other in the butt when necessary.

**HOW RUNNING CHANGED MY LIFE:** The most rewarding part of running is the confidence I have gained in all aspects of my life. I am proud of myself and my accomplishments, and cherish the wonderful friends I have made in the running community. Three years ago I would have never imagined I'd be a two-time marathoner. Running, whether I'm training for a race or just going for a quick jog, will always be a part of my life.

**I WISH I'D KNOWN:** Trust yourself and push yourself. I've learned that physical activity is more of a mental challenge than anything—it's amazing what the body can do when you put your mind to something. Being a runner is something truly special; it takes guts. Build a support group of friends and create a goal rather than just "I want to get in shape." Creating a goal, such as signing up for a 5-K, will encourage you to keep up with a routine.

# FOR BEGINNERS ONLY

**Q** How do you start running—or return to it—if you have health issues?

**A** It is always best to consult with your doctor before beginning any exercise program, but it is especially important when you have known medical issues. Your health care professional will probably have some guidelines to follow. He or she may even refer you to a sports medicine professional or a physical therapist for additional assistance.

There are three very important fitness components to all exercise programs that you can control: frequency, intensity, and duration. Frequency means how often you exercise, intensity refers to how hard you exercise, and duration is the length of each exercise session. Manipulating these components is the basis of all training plans. If given the green light to exercise, and specifically to walk or run, begin conservatively. The length or duration of your exercise sessions depends upon your current fitness level. A short workout—say 15 minutes of walking—may be plenty, initially. Keep in mind that exercise should invigorate you and leave you feeling energized and exhilarated, not exhausted or in pain. For frequency, begin with 2 or 3 days a week. Exercising every other day automatically builds in recovery time between workouts. It also gives you time to assess how you feel afterward. Note any aches, pains, or discomfort. Dial it back if you notice any of these signs. What about the intensity of the workout? How fast or hard should you run or walk? This will also depend on your current level of fitness.

You might monitor your intensity by using the Talk Test, which states that you should be able to talk or hold a conversation while exercising. If you cannot talk in complete sentances—say you're exercising so intensely that you can only get a few words out—the intensity is too high, slow it down. On the other hand, if you can sing while exercising, you need to pick up the pace.

If you have your physician's approval to transition to running, after several weeks of walking, incorporate short run intervals of 30 seconds into your regular works. You can gradually lengthen the run interval as your fitness allows. Most important, though, don't overdo it. Monitor how you feel during and after each exercise session and use this as your guide for the next workout.

You might also consider starting your walking or running program on a treadmill. The treadmill surface is also more forgiving than the road or sidewalk so the impact will be a bit gentler on your body. The base on the treadmill gives more than asphalt, concrete, or brick so it's a good place to begin. And if you experience any issues during your workout and need to stop immediately, you are in a safe environment protected from the outside elements. When or if you transition to walking or running outdoors, you will need additional conditioning time for toughening up muscles and bones for these harder surfaces.

*Coach and exercise physiologist Susan Paul, author of "For Beginners Only" column,* Runner's World, *is program manager for the Track Shack Foundation. Paul has coached is program director for the Orlando Track Shack Foundation. For more information, visit trackshack.com.*

## NUTRITION

Plain water is the best way to go. But if you just can't stomach it, try one of the many flavored, calorie-free waters on the market. Be sure to read the nutrition label and avoid extra calories and sugar. If you want a natural option that's a little tastier, try adding a slice of orange, lemon, lime, grapefruit; a few mint leaves; or even cucumber to your water.

"I am a firm believer in getting off one's butt and running. For me it isn't about the speed or the distance necessarily, it's just getting dressed and going out to run."

—**WILL STARR,** runner, Swarthmore, Pennsylvania, runnersworld.com/will-starr

## MONDAY

Route:

Distance: Time:

NOTES:

Cross-training:

## TUESDAY

Route:

Distance: Time:

NOTES:

Cross-training:

## WEDNESDAY

Route:

Distance: Time:

NOTES:

Cross-training:

## THURSDAY

Route:

Distance: Time:

NOTES:

Cross-training:

## FRIDAY

Route:

Distance: Time:

NOTES:

Cross-training:

## SATURDAY

Route:

Distance: Time:

NOTES:

Cross-training:

## SUNDAY

Route:

Distance: Time:

NOTES:

Cross-training:

## NOTES

WEEKLY MILEAGE TOTAL:

TOTAL MILEAGE TO DATE:

## INJURY

During the summer, you're at a higher risk for chafing. Skin-to-skin and skin-to-clothing rubbing can cause this red, raw rash that can bleed, sting, and make you yelp during your postrun shower. To prevent it, wear moisture-wicking, seamless, tagless gear. Apply Vaseline, sports lube, Band-Aids, or NipGuards before you run. To treat chafing, wash the area with soap and water, apply an antibacterial ointment, and cover with a bandage.

## TRAINING

To lower your risk of sunburn, avoid running between 10 a.m. and 4 p.m., wear a hat, run in the shade, and wear a broad-spectrum sunscreen with an SPF of 30 or higher. Reapply it every hour that you're outside. Apply it 20 minutes before you head outside.

## NUTRITION

Remember: Just because a bread is brown doesn't mean that it's whole grain. Look for labels that say 100 percent whole grain, or look for these terms on the list of ingredients: whole grain, whole wheat, stoneground whole oats, and oatmeal. If you see terms like enriched flour, bran, or wheat germ, chances are the bread isn't whole grain.

"The journey isn't always perfect, but always worth taking."

—**KARA GOUCHER**, Olympic marathoner

### MONDAY
Route:

Distance: Time:

NOTES:

Cross-training:

### TUESDAY
Route:

Distance: Time:

NOTES:

Cross-training:

### WEDNESDAY
Route:

Distance: Time:

NOTES:

Cross-training:

### THURSDAY
Route:

Distance: Time:

NOTES:

Cross-training:

### FRIDAY
Route:

Distance: Time:

NOTES:

Cross-training:

## SATURDAY

Route:

Distance: Time:

NOTES:

Cross-training:

## SUNDAY

Route:

Distance: Time:

NOTES:

Cross-training:

## NOTES

WEEKLY MILEAGE TOTAL:

TOTAL MILEAGE TO DATE:

### INJURY

When running in the heat, if you start to feel unwell—whether you have a headache, feel nauseous, or the workout just feels harder than usual—always back off. Don't try to push through it. If you're running easy, walk. If you're walking, then stop and get in the shade.

### TRAINING

At a stop sign or light, always assume that the driver or cyclist does not see you. Wait for the oncoming motorist to wave you through—then acknowledge with your own polite wave. Use hand signals (as you would on a bicycle) to show which way you plan to turn.

## NUTRITION

Stay hydrated throughout the day. This is the best way to avoid a last-minute push to pound fluids before a workout, a sloshy or nauseous feeling while you're on the road, and unwanted pit stops on your run. So sip small amounts of water or calorie-free beverages between and with meals.

"A winner is a person who goes out today and every day and attempts to be the best runner and best person he can be. Winning is about struggle and effort and optimism, and never, ever, ever giving up."

—**AMBY BURFOOT,** 1968 Boston Marathon winner, *Runner's World* editor at large

## MONDAY

Route:

Distance: Time:

NOTES:

Cross-training:

## TUESDAY

Route:

Distance: Time:

NOTES:

Cross-training:

## WEDNESDAY

Route:

Distance: Time:

NOTES:

Cross-training:

## THURSDAY

Route:

Distance: Time:

NOTES:

Cross-training:

## FRIDAY

Route:

Distance: Time:

NOTES:

Cross-training:

## SATURDAY

Route:

Distance: Time:

NOTES:

Cross-training:

## SUNDAY

Route:

Distance: Time:

NOTES:

Cross-training:

## NOTES

WEEKLY MILEAGE TOTAL:

TOTAL MILEAGE TO DATE:

## INJURY

Before you start working out in the heat, make sure that you've been exercising regularly for 4 to 6 weeks first. The heat is another stress on the body, just like exercise. As you get in shape, you are going to withstand the heat better.

## TRAINING

Cross-training with cycling, swimming, the elliptical trainer, or the rowing machine can play an important role in your overall fitness routine. It gives the muscles you use in walking and running a chance to recover while strengthening other parts of the body, boosting all-around fitness, and preventing injuries. Plus it helps prevent burnout. It can take a while to develop the strength and the know-how to get a good workout. So make it a regular part of your routine from the beginning. If you wait until you're forced to cross-train because of poor weather or injury, you might not get a good workout.

WEEK 28 WEEK OF ____ TO ____

## NUTRITION

When you're adequately hydrated, your urine will be the color of pale lemonade or straw. If it's clear, you're drinking too much. If it's the color of apple juice, drink more.

"Running can open so many doors; improved health, new social groups, a sense of accomplishment, the list goes on. What I have found is that the key to success is consistency. Just get out there and run, and in no time you will be doing things that you never thought possible."

—DOUGLAS D'ADABIE, runner, Port-of-Spain, Trinidad and Tobago, runnersworld.com/douglas-dadabie

### MONDAY

Route:

Distance: Time:

NOTES:

Cross-training:

### TUESDAY

Route:

Distance: Time:

NOTES:

Cross-training:

### WEDNESDAY

Route:

Distance: Time:

NOTES:

Cross-training:

### THURSDAY

Route:

Distance: Time:

NOTES:

Cross-training:

### FRIDAY

Route:

Distance: Time:

NOTES:

Cross-training:

## SATURDAY

Route:

Distance: Time:

NOTES:

Cross-training:

## SUNDAY

Route:

Distance: Time:

NOTES:

Cross-training:

## NOTES

WEEKLY MILEAGE TOTAL:

TOTAL MILEAGE TO DATE:

### INJURY

Watch out for any aches or pains that persist or worsen as you run or prompt you to change your gait. Each person has his or her own unique orthopedic threshold for how many miles they can log and how fast they can go before getting injured. That's determined by a person's unique genetics, anatomy, biomechanics, and history of injury.

### TRAINING

Cross-training can provide an excellent cardio workout with zero impact and strengthens muscles that running neglects. But if you do the activity wrong, you could get hurt. Before you hit the machines on your own, meet with a trainer to get tips on proper form and appropriate weight levels to start with. Many gyms offer a few free sessions to new members.

WEEK 29 WEEK OF TO

## NUTRITION

If you are refueling on the road with an energy gel, be sure to wash down those carbs with a sip of water. Do not chase an energy gel, chew, or any carb-heavy fuel with sports drinks, which have carbs, too. Doing so dumps too many carbs into your gut at once and is likely to send you dashing for the nearest toilet.

"The long runs . . . are a genuine adventure for me—a physical challenge in an otherwise mostly cerebral, abstract sort of daily life. And you don't have to go to a mountain or anything. It starts right out the front door of your home."

—**JOHN WALTER,** runner, Ankeny, Iowa, runnersworld.com/john-walter

### MONDAY

Route:

Distance: Time:

NOTES:

Cross-training:

### TUESDAY

Route:

Distance: Time:

NOTES:

Cross-training:

### WEDNESDAY

Route:

Distance: Time:

NOTES:

Cross-training:

### THURSDAY

Route:

Distance: Time:

NOTES:

Cross-training:

### FRIDAY

Route:

Distance: Time:

NOTES:

Cross-training:

## SATURDAY

Route:

Distance: Time:

NOTES:

Cross-training:

## SUNDAY

Route:

Distance: Time:

NOTES:

Cross-training:

## NOTES

WEEKLY MILEAGE TOTAL:

TOTAL MILEAGE TO DATE:

### INJURY

Give yourself time to adjust to the heat. It can take 7 to 10 exercise sessions over the course of 2 weeks to adjust to the heat. But even then, don't do the hardest workout in the hottest time of day. Run in the early morning or late at night, or work out inside.

### TRAINING

Pace and heart rate don't really translate from running to cross-training activities. So it's best to do any given activity—cycling, swimming, elliptical, or rowing machine—for the same amount of time that you'd spend running at the same level of effort. So if you'd normally run or walk for 30 minutes at an easy effort, substitute 30 minutes on the elliptical at an easy effort.

# WEEK 30 WEEK OF ____ TO ____

## NUTRITION

Many sports drinks look appealing, but they are also laden with calories and sugar, which makes it easy to consume all the calories that you worked so hard to burn. Avoid specialty coffee drinks, high-octane sports drinks, and even fruit juice, all of which can be high in calories.

"Believe that you can run farther or faster. Believe that you're young enough, old enough, strong enough, and so on to accomplish everything you want to do. Don't let worn-out beliefs stop you from moving beyond yourself."

—**JOHN BINGHAM,** running speaker and writer

## MONDAY

**Route:**

**Distance:** **Time:**

**NOTES:**

**Cross-training:**

## TUESDAY

**Route:**

**Distance:** **Time:**

**NOTES:**

**Cross-training:**

## WEDNESDAY

**Route:**

**Distance:** **Time:**

**NOTES:**

**Cross-training:**

## THURSDAY

**Route:**

**Distance:** **Time:**

**NOTES:**

**Cross-training:**

## FRIDAY

**Route:**

**Distance:** **Time:**

**NOTES:**

**Cross-training:**

## SATURDAY

Route:

Distance: Time:

NOTES:

Cross-training:

## SUNDAY

Route:

Distance: Time:

NOTES:

Cross-training:

## NOTES

WEEKLY MILEAGE TOTAL:

TOTAL MILEAGE TO DATE:

### INJURY

Hydration becomes most important during intense exercise in the heat. Even slight dehydration can make the effort feel tougher. So drink extra water and electrolytes when it's hot and humid outside. The best bet for rehydration is to consume a low-cal beverage that contains electrolytes such as sodium and potassium. Good choices include sports drinks, coconut water, or water with a slice of fruit. The refreshing hint of flavor may drive you to drink more.

### TRAINING

If the workout feels harder than it usually does, take some time to check your breathing. It's very common to hold the breath when the going gets tough, without even realizing it. And that makes the effort feel much tougher than it needs to.

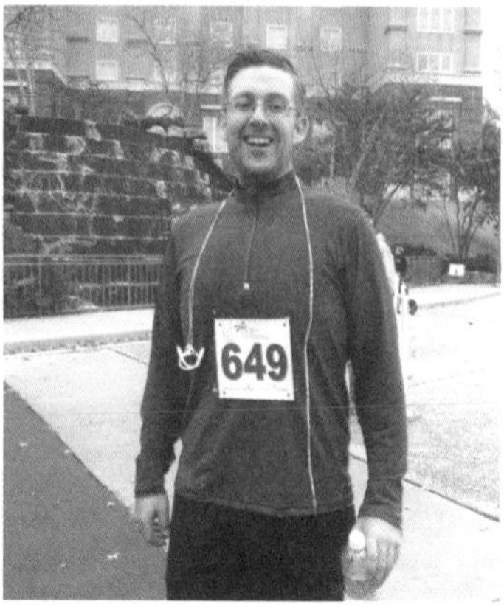


# B. J. KEETON

College English instructor and sci-fi/fantasy author
Lawrenceburg, Tennessee

**WHAT GOT ME GOING:** My wife and I went to an amusement park and the attendant could barely click the safety harness of the roller coaster over my gut—and I was in the plus-size seat. I thought I was going to fall out of the seat. I couldn't let my weight—which I had never cared about that much before—hold me back from living my life. I was 27 years old and a newlywed. I had my whole life in front of me. I needed to be able to enjoy it.

**SECRET OF MY SUCCESS:** I downloaded the Couch-to-5-K app. It wanted me to run for 60 seconds at a time, and I just couldn't do it. So I walked until my lungs were able to handle the strain and then started the Couch-to-5-K program. I was diagnosed with exercise-induced asthma (EIA) and that, combined with my inherent laziness, was almost a death sentence for me. After reading online about runners overcoming EIA, I talked to my doctor, and he didn't think there'd be anything wrong with me puffing on Albuterol before a run. Since then, I take my hit after I lace up, and I'm pretty much good to go. I always tell people that you can't necessarily beat having asthma, but you sure can outrun it.

**HOW RUNNING CHANGED MY LIFE:** At my heaviest, I weighed 310 pounds, and right now, I'm 164. I've lost 146 pounds, and that's more than I ever thought possible. So I kept milestone goals (250, 220, 200) that were both realistic and far enough away that I had to keep working myself to reach them. I saw each pound as another few months alive, with my wife and my family, doing the stuff I love to do. I never thought it was possible for my body to be this size or this shape. I mean, I love having people (even family members!) not recognize me in public, or being able to walk in a store and buy clothes I like without having to special order them. And I love the running community: People are friendly and happy and delightfully inclusive.

**I WISH I'D KNOWN:** It gets better. Really. I promise. The hurting stops. The exhaustion goes away. The fatigue and cramps and blisters and all of that are temporary. I know it doesn't seem that way, and I know that you feel like you want to die after 30 seconds, but it eventually becomes one of the best things in the world. But you have to stick with it.

# FOR BEGINNERS ONLY

**Q** I'm following a training plan but I missed a workout. What do I do?

**A** When you have a training plan with specific workouts, they are intended to build upon one another, so it is important to do them in sequence. Rest days allow the body time to recover from a workout and time for adaptation to occur from the physical stresses being placed upon it. The rest period and adaptation are part of what makes you fitter, faster, or stronger and able to meet the demands of the next workout.

When something, like life, interferes with your training plan and you must miss a workout, you have some options. If you can't workout at all, count that day as a rest day. Move the workout to the next day, but keep the same number of specified recovery days between that workout and the next one. This means moving your next workout too. If you're following a training plan, this will throw you off the plan a bit, but you are keeping the same progression and the same recovery intact. Pushing workouts too close together increases your risk of injury, so it's better to have an extra day or two of rest. However, if it turns into more than a day or two off, then you need to re-evaluate the plan because you risk de-training and increasing your risk of injury.

Another option is to do a short, easy run to maintain your current fitness level when you can't fit in a specific workout. Doing something is better than nothing and this will help keep you focused on your long-term goals. Then, do the specific workout as soon as possible, keeping the same number of recovery days after the workout before moving on to the next workout.

And, yet another option is to put your training plan on hold, maintain your fitness level, and then resume your training plan when life settles down. This doesn't mean become a couch potato! But, rather maintain the fitness level you have accomplished to date until you can return to following your training plan, uninterrupted, again. Short, easy runs allow runners to maintain their fitness through hectic times and then resume training when life is more manageable. Running should serve as a stress outlet rather than a stress creator so if you feel bad about missing workouts, simply put your training plan on hold and enjoy some guilt-free running until you can resume more serious training.

When life gets hectic, it helps to plan ahead. Look at your upcoming week and set your workouts in line with what is realistic for you to accomplish given that week's demands. By planning out the week, you may find you can enjoy the work and family activities, the workouts, and the rest days! It's important that running and fitness goals are in sync with real life too.

*Coach and exercise physiologist Susan Paul, author of "For Beginners Only" column,* Runner's World, *is program manager for the Track Shack Foundation. Paul has coached is program director for the Orlando Track Shack Foundation. For more information, visit trackshack.com.*

## NUTRITION

A variety of sports drinks and energy gels and chews are on the market. Figure out what you like and what sits well with you. Some people can't stomach anything solid and choose to rely on sports drinks, which can have 15 to 30 grams of carbs per 16 ounces. Each product has its own unique blend of sugar and other ingredients, so try as many different kinds as you can. If you're training for a race, try the brand that will be offered at aid stations at the race to determine if that works for you.

"My long-term goal is to be around to run long-term."

—**JEREMY DOBRICK,** runner and cancer survivor, New York City, runnersworld.com/jeremy-dobrick

### MONDAY

Route:

Distance: Time:

NOTES:

Cross-training:

### TUESDAY

Route:

Distance: Time:

NOTES:

Cross-training:

### WEDNESDAY

Route:

Distance: Time:

NOTES:

Cross-training:

### THURSDAY

Route:

Distance: Time:

NOTES:

Cross-training:

### FRIDAY

Route:

Distance: Time:

NOTES:

Cross-training:

## SATURDAY

Route:

Distance: Time:

NOTES:

Cross-training:

## SUNDAY

Route:

Distance: Time:

NOTES:

Cross-training:

## NOTES

WEEKLY MILEAGE TOTAL:

TOTAL MILEAGE TO DATE:

### INJURY

Starting a running program is also a great time to start working on your core strength, particularly your glutes and abdominal muscles. A strong core makes it easier to stay upright—even when you're tired—and avoid leaning too far forward from your hip, which can lead to injury.

### TRAINING

Run for the hills, not away from them. Hills build leg and lung strength and give you the foundation of fitness you need to get faster on the track. As you go uphill, try to stay relaxed. Keep your gaze straight ahead, your shoulders down, and envision your feet pushing up and off the leg, and the road rising to meet you. Try to maintain an even level of effort as you're climbing up the hill and as you're making your descent. Avoid trying to charge the hill; you don't want to be spent by the time you get to the top.

WEEK 32 WEEK OF ______ TO ______

## NUTRITION

As you try out fuel during your training runs, keep track of what you took and how you felt afterward. Did you get a burst of energy? Or did you feel sluggish? Were you able to keep your pace constant but then hit the wall toward the end of the workout? Did the fuel tie your stomach in knots? Or did it sit well?

"Success is peace of mind, which is a direct result of self-satisfaction in knowing you did your best to become the best that you are capable of becoming."

—**JOHN WOODEN,** American basketball player and coach

## MONDAY

**Route:**

**Distance:** **Time:**

**NOTES:**

**Cross-training:**

## TUESDAY

**Route:**

**Distance:** **Time:**

**NOTES:**

**Cross-training:**

## WEDNESDAY

**Route:**

**Distance:** **Time:**

**NOTES:**

**Cross-training:**

## THURSDAY

**Route:**

**Distance:** **Time:**

**NOTES:**

**Cross-training:**

## FRIDAY

**Route:**

**Distance:** **Time:**

**NOTES:**

**Cross-training:**

## SATURDAY

Route:

Distance: Time:

NOTES:

Cross-training:

## SUNDAY

Route:

Distance: Time:

NOTES:

Cross-training:

## NOTES

WEEKLY MILEAGE TOTAL:

TOTAL MILEAGE TO DATE:

### INJURY

When going up a hill, keep your head and chest up. Look straight ahead. Visualize the road rising to meet you. Keep your shoulders back. Push up and off the hill, springing from your toes. Don't bend at the waist and hunch over. Keep your hands and fists loose.

### TRAINING

Try different kinds of cross-training activities until you find the one that works best for you. Once you find it, stick with it. Once you become more comfortable on it, you can boost your heart rate and get a good sweat going. Sticking with one activity also makes it easier for you to track your progress. Each time you can more fairly compare one workout to the next.

## NUTRITION

When you're regularly working out and trying to shed pounds, it's a good idea to check in with the scale once a week, to see progress or to stop a landslide before it starts.

## MONDAY

Route:

Distance: Time:

NOTES:

Cross-training:

## TUESDAY

Route:

Distance: Time:

NOTES:

Cross-training:

## WEDNESDAY

Route:

Distance: Time:

NOTES:

Cross-training:

## THURSDAY

Route:

Distance: Time:

NOTES:

Cross-training:

## FRIDAY

Route:

Distance: Time:

NOTES:

Cross-training:

"Run in places you love with people you like. Enjoying your surroundings and training partners will strengthen your commitment to running and bring out the best in you."

—**DEENA KASTOR,** Olympic marathoner

## SATURDAY

Route:

Distance: Time:

NOTES:

Cross-training:

## SUNDAY

Route:

Distance: Time:

NOTES:

Cross-training:

## NOTES

WEEKLY MILEAGE TOTAL:

TOTAL MILEAGE TO DATE:

### INJURY

When running downhill, watch your form. Keep your torso upright. Look straight ahead. Visualize controlled falling. Keep your nose over your toes. Step softly; don't let your feet slap the pavement. Avoid leaning back and braking with the quads. That will put you at risk for injury.

### TRAINING

Want to track your fitness gains? Take your heart rate for 1 minute first thing in the morning before you get out of bed. Put two fingers on your pulse and time the number of beats per minute. Write the number down in your training log. As you get fitter, your resting heart rate will get lower. That's because your heart is getting stronger, so it doesn't have to make as many beats to pump the blood that your body needs. When your heart rate gets lower, you know that your body is responding to the training and getting more fit.

WEEK 34 WEEK OF TO

## NUTRITION

It's okay to drink coffee or caffeinated tea before a workout. In fact studies have shown that caffeine boosts energy and alertness. Just be sure to leave enough time between your java and your run to hit the bathroom. The heat of the liquid gets the bowels moving, and you don't want to have to make an unwanted stop on the run.

"Running has taught me that we are capable of doing more than we ever imagined, that we can overcome huge obstacles, and that consistency pays off!"

—**AMY PEAVY-SMITH,** runner, Athens, Georgia, runnersworld.com/amy-peavy-smith

### MONDAY

Route:

Distance: Time:

NOTES:

Cross-training:

### TUESDAY

Route:

Distance: Time:

NOTES:

Cross-training:

### WEDNESDAY

Route:

Distance: Time:

NOTES:

Cross-training:

### THURSDAY

Route:

Distance: Time:

NOTES:

Cross-training:

### FRIDAY

Route:

Distance: Time:

NOTES:

Cross-training:

## SATURDAY

Route:

Distance: Time:

NOTES:

Cross-training:

## SUNDAY

Route:

Distance: Time:

NOTES:

Cross-training:

## NOTES

WEEKLY MILEAGE TOTAL:

TOTAL MILEAGE TO DATE:

## INJURY

If you are injured, see a sports medicine doctor who can determine what the problem is and prescribe some physical therapy. If the problem is linked to your running form, you might consider seeing a running clinic with a biomechanist, where someone can evaluate your running gait, strength, and flexibility. He or she can suggest footwear that offers the support you need, plus exercises to help offset any muscle imbalances.

## TRAINING

When you're at the track, leave the headphones at home. When you are close to fatigued runners in a confined space trying to hit top speed, you'll want to tune in to what's going on around you.

WEEK 35 WEEK OF TO

## NUTRITION

So often we're eating not to soothe a growling stomach but to relieve boredom, anxiety, stress, sadness, or some other emotion. So find a solution that eases your discomfort without leaving you with extra pounds (and the guilt). Go outside, knit, weed the garden, write a letter, call a friend, listen to music, or just leave the kitchen so food will be out of sight. On the fridge or the pantry, keep a list of safe alternatives to eating that you can refer to whenever a snack attack takes hold.

"I saw hundreds of sunrises—each one more magnificent than the one before. I started exploring trails and lost the fear of getting lost. I ran hills, and began to wonder what lay over the horizon."

—**VANESSA RUNS,** author of *The Summit Seeker*

### MONDAY

Route:

Distance: Time:

NOTES:

Cross-training:

### TUESDAY

Route:

Distance: Time:

NOTES:

Cross-training:

### WEDNESDAY

Route:

Distance: Time:

NOTES:

Cross-training:

### THURSDAY

Route:

Distance: Time:

NOTES:

Cross-training:

### FRIDAY

Route:

Distance: Time:

NOTES:

Cross-training:

## SATURDAY

Route:

Distance: Time:

NOTES:

Cross-training:

## SUNDAY

Route:

Distance: Time:

NOTES:

Cross-training:

## NOTES

WEEKLY MILEAGE TOTAL:

TOTAL MILEAGE TO DATE:

## INJURY

Anytime you run on a new type of surface, expect some new aches and pains. Your muscles, joints, and ligaments will be worked in new ways that they aren't when you're pounding pavement. So you may feel a little soreness in the 2 days after the workout, particularly in your ankles, calf muscles, or shins.

## TRAINING

When you're running on trails, look ahead. To find the best footing, keep your eyes on the trail a few steps ahead of you. Shorten your stride. And forget about pace. It's best to focus on level of effort. With different footing and an unfamiliar route, your pace will slow. Slow down as much as you need to avoid falling. With the uneven and new surface, you'll still get a great workout.

# WEEK 36 WEEK OF ______ TO ______

## NUTRITION

You know that exercise burns calories while you're working out, but the burn continues even after you stop. Studies have shown that regular exercise boosts "afterburn"—that is, the number of calories you burn after exercise. And you don't have to be sprinting at lightning speed to get this benefit. This happens when you're exercising at an intensity that's a little faster than your easy pace.

"My vote for the smartest running streak goes to the annual-mileage streak. Try to hit 1,000 miles a year for as long as you can. That's roughly 20 miles a week, a solid marker of dedication and persistence. Annual mileage streaks give you a bar to clear, but also give you wiggle room for flu, injuries, new jobs, new kids, new relationships, new homes, and all the usual stuff."

—**AMBY BURFOOT**, 1968 Boston Marathon winner, *Runner's World* editor at large

## MONDAY

Route:

Distance: Time:

NOTES:

Cross-training:

## TUESDAY

Route:

Distance: Time:

NOTES:

Cross-training:

## WEDNESDAY

Route:

Distance: Time:

NOTES:

Cross-training:

## THURSDAY

Route:

Distance: Time:

NOTES:

Cross-training:

## FRIDAY

Route:

Distance: Time:

NOTES:

Cross-training:

## SATURDAY

Route:

Distance: Time:

NOTES:

Cross-training:

## SUNDAY

Route:

Distance: Time:

NOTES:

Cross-training:

## NOTES

WEEKLY MILEAGE TOTAL:

TOTAL MILEAGE TO DATE:

### INJURY

When you're going downhill, it's easy to fly and enjoy feeling gravity's pull. But steep descents can tax your muscles even more than big climbs. Running downhill can generate more force (and soreness) than running uphill or on level ground. To reduce risk of injury, and strengthen your muscles for downhill running, start by practicing running downhill at an easy pace on soft surfaces like grass.

### TRAINING

Freshen up your routine every few weeks by running for a certain duration of time instead of miles.

## MELISSA PEARSON

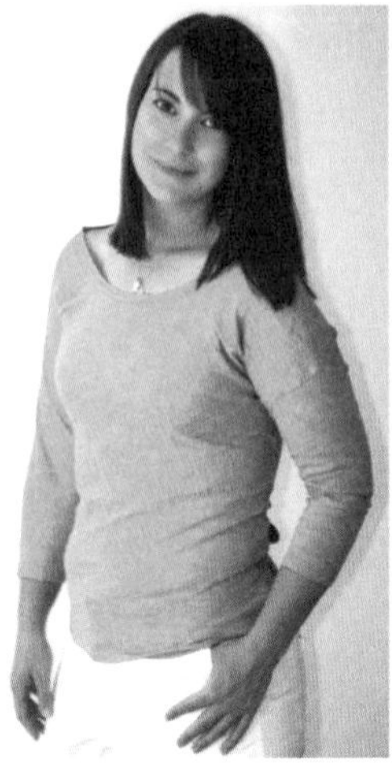

Athletic trainer
Terre Haute, Indiana

**WHAT GOT ME GOING:** I was very overweight and needed to lose about 80 pounds. I was a college athlete, and it was depressing to see what I'd let myself become. I began with a walking plan. Over time, I progressed to run/walk with the *Runner's World* Start Running plan. Then I added in yoga and body-weight strength exercise a few days a week.

**SECRET OF MY SUCCESS:** The most difficult challenge for me is to not give up when a run is not going as well as planned. I've always had a tendency to quit when the going gets tough. When I started running, I made two rules: (1) Not giving up on a run unless I truly am in trouble (overheated, injured) and (2) if I did give up on a run, I have to repeat that entire week of the training plan. The prospect of having to step back makes me truly evaluate what's happening and whether or not I am really needing to stop, or just giving up.

**HOW RUNNING CHANGED MY LIFE:** The biggest reward has been proving to myself that I really can do something that seemed impossible at first. Six months ago I couldn't fathom running a minute without stopping! I started at 215 pounds, and my goal weight is 135. I'm currently at 145 . . . almost there!

I obsessively measure, weigh, count, whatever, everything I put in my mouth. My digital food scale is my best friend. I honestly don't know how people lose weight without one! I was going out to eat too often, and eating huge portions in general. I started taking lunch to work, eating small snacks, and properly portioning serving sizes. I wasn't eating all that unhealthily before; I was just eating so much. Now my portions are reasonable.

**I WISH I'D KNOWN:** Go slow. All the times I failed an exercise program were because I went gung-ho right away and got sore and burned out. Start with walking or something else completely achievable. Your progress will snowball into success.

# FOR BEGINNERS ONLY

**Q** I'm a new runner. Is it okay to run on a track? Or is it just for faster veteran runners?

**A** The track may seem like it's just for fast veteran runners, but it's actually a perfect place for new runners to start working out. After all, it's flat, traffic-free, and the distance is measured.

If you haven't been to the track since grade school don't be daunted. There are just a few track manners that you'll need to mind.

- Most tracks are 400 meters–or one quarter mile around, so four laps around is about one mile.
- Be sure to run counterclockwise on the track so you don't collide with oncoming runners.
- Leave the headphones at home so you can hear people approaching from behind.
- Steer clear of lane one, as that's where those who are doing speed workouts tend to be.

Don't feel like you have to run fast at the track. But after you've been running regularly for awhile, say about 6 weeks, you may want to try speed workouts. These workouts, which involve running specific intervals of time or distance at a faster pace, can help you develop stronger legs and lungs. But most important, they can keep your exercise regime from getting stale.

The workout below is a great place to start. This helps you get your body and mind accustomed to picking up the pace for short periods of time. The short intervals make the bouts of hard work seem doable. With each walk break you have a chance to recover enough for your next bout of hard work.

## Straights and Curves

- Walk for 5 minutes to warmup.
- Then run the straight stretches of the track and walk the curves.
- Repeat that cycle twice.
- Leave water at a spot that you can drink after you finish each loop.
- On the run segment, get into a rhythm that's comfortable, but don't sprint.

You can also do this workout on the road. Use different landmarks to mark your intervals. You might run to a tree, mailbox, telephone pole, or stop sign. Then walk. Once you catch your breath, pick another landmark to run to. Then walk to recover. Repeat the cycle two or three times.

*Coach and exercise physiologist Susan Paul, author of "For Beginners Only" column,* Runner's World, *is program manager for the Track Shack Foundation. Paul has coached is program director for the Orlando Track Shack Foundation. For more information, visit trackshack.com.*

# WEEK 37 WEEK OF ______ TO ______

## NUTRITION

Avoid weighing yourself multiple times a day. Your weight can fluctuate wildly throughout the day, depending on how much you drank, the amount of sodium you've consumed, and how much fat, protein, or carbs you've had.

"If you're a runner and you're around older runners, you just get the sense of what's possible. You have no clue, if you're by yourself, how fast you can run. You have no sense of what your limits are."

—MALCOLM GLADWELL, author of *Outliers* and *The Tipping Point*

## MONDAY

Route:

Distance: Time:

NOTES:

Cross-training:

## TUESDAY

Route:

Distance: Time:

NOTES:

Cross-training:

## WEDNESDAY

Route:

Distance: Time:

NOTES:

Cross-training:

## THURSDAY

Route:

Distance: Time:

NOTES:

Cross-training:

## FRIDAY

Route:

Distance: Time:

NOTES:

Cross-training:

## SATURDAY

Route:

Distance: Time:

NOTES:

Cross-training:

## SUNDAY

Route:

Distance: Time:

NOTES:

Cross-training:

## NOTES

WEEKLY MILEAGE TOTAL:

TOTAL MILEAGE TO DATE:

### INJURY

Listen to your body. Most running injuries don't just come out of nowhere and blindside you. Usually, there are warning signs—aches, soreness, and persistent pain. It's up to you to heed those signs. If you don't, you could hurt something else as you try to change your gait to compensate for the pain.

### TRAINING

Runners tend to be hyperaware of their bodies, self-medicating with ice or ibuprofen to treat aches and pains. But minor injuries could turn into serious ones. Instead, see a doctor sooner rather than later. If the pain has lingered for 3 days, schedule an appointment.

# WEEK 38 WEEK OF ____ TO ____

## NUTRITION

While there are a ton of engineered sports foods on the market, a lot of more traditional foods can offer the same boost—without the unwanted side effects. Jelly packets have 13 grams of carbs per packet and provide two types of sugar. Gumdrops contain about 4 grams of carbs per candy. Take 10 with you for midrun energy.

"The perfect run? When it's an hour later and I don't want to stop and I feel energized. I walk back into my house with sort of a happy buzz, and I feel psyched to take the garbage out. I can do all of this stuff. All of the mundane stuff that can get on your nerves seems like an easy thing to do. It's not like I suddenly do something different, but the stuff that I am doing seems much more manageable and fun."

—JULIE BOWEN,
actress, *Modern Family*

## MONDAY

Route:

Distance: Time:

NOTES:

Cross-training:

## TUESDAY

Route:

Distance: Time:

NOTES:

Cross-training:

## WEDNESDAY

Route:

Distance: Time:

NOTES:

Cross-training:

## THURSDAY

Route:

Distance: Time:

NOTES:

Cross-training:

## FRIDAY

Route:

Distance: Time:

NOTES:

Cross-training:

## SATURDAY

Route:

Distance: Time:

NOTES:

Cross-training:

## SUNDAY

Route:

Distance: Time:

NOTES:

Cross-training:

## NOTES

WEEKLY MILEAGE TOTAL:

TOTAL MILEAGE TO DATE:

### INJURY

Some muscle soreness is to be expected anytime you are pushing your body farther or faster than it's accustomed to going. But there are some pains that you shouldn't ignore. Any sharp pains or pains that persist or worsen as you walk, run, or go about your daily activities are signals to rest for 2–3 days and see a doctor. Also, beware of any pains that are only on one side of the body.

### TRAINING

When you hit the track, run counterclockwise. And steer clear of lane one, the innermost lane of the track. If you're warming up, cooling down, or running slower, move to an outer lane.

WEEK 39 WEEK OF ______ TO ______

## NUTRITION

Want to eat less without feeling deprived? Use smaller plates. If you always serve dinner on a dinner plate, you're bound to fill it up and ask for seconds. Choose a smaller plate and you won't be able to pile on quite as many calories.

"Running makes me feel calm, happy, and good about my body. It makes me feel good to have done something for myself that day. It really helps on the inside and outside."

—**DANICA PATRICK,** professional race-car driver

### MONDAY

Route:

Distance: Time:

NOTES:

Cross-training:

### TUESDAY

Route:

Distance: Time:

NOTES:

Cross-training:

### WEDNESDAY

Route:

Distance: Time:

NOTES:

Cross-training:

### THURSDAY

Route:

Distance: Time:

NOTES:

Cross-training:

### FRIDAY

Route:

Distance: Time:

NOTES:

Cross-training:

## SATURDAY

Route:

Distance: Time:

NOTES:

Cross-training:

## SUNDAY

Route:

Distance: Time:

NOTES:

Cross-training:

## NOTES

WEEKLY MILEAGE TOTAL:

TOTAL MILEAGE TO DATE:

### INJURY

Lots of people get hung up on running a certain number of miles per week, and if they miss a day or two, try to cram in extra miles. Going from a little running to a lot in short order is a recipe for disaster. Stick to the training plan as best you can, but when life gets in the way—or you feel fatigued or sore—it's okay to put the workout off until another day, or skip it altogether.

### TRAINING

It's easy to fall into a rut of doing the same route, day after day. If you do, after a while the hills won't feel as challenging. So incorporate a variety of short, steep climbs and long, gradual inclines. The shorter climbs at higher intensity will give you a quick cardiovascular boost and help improve your aerobic capacity. The longer climbs at an easier effort will help build your endurance.

## NUTRITION

If you're curious to see how much fluid you lose during an hour-long workout, here's how to find out: Weigh yourself naked before a workout, then again after you're done. If you lost 1 pound during the workout, you sweated 16 ounces (1 pound). Next time, when you're working out in similar conditions, try to take in 16 ounces of fluids during the workout to replace what you lost through sweating.

"I would tell anyone who wants to run but is embarrassed to go to a 5-K and see what it's all about! You'll see people of all sizes. You don't have to run it—even if you walk it, you'll realize what a supportive community the running world is. We are all nervous at our first race."

—**ALISON SWEENEY,** host of *The Biggest Loser*

### MONDAY

**Route:**

**Distance:** **Time:**

**NOTES:**

**Cross-training:**

### TUESDAY

**Route:**

**Distance:** **Time:**

**NOTES:**

**Cross-training:**

### WEDNESDAY

**Route:**

**Distance:** **Time:**

**NOTES:**

**Cross-training:**

### THURSDAY

**Route:**

**Distance:** **Time:**

**NOTES:**

**Cross-training:**

### FRIDAY

**Route:**

**Distance:** **Time:**

**NOTES:**

**Cross-training:**

## SATURDAY

Route:

Distance: Time:

NOTES:

Cross-training:

## SUNDAY

Route:

Distance: Time:

NOTES:

Cross-training:

## NOTES

WEEKLY MILEAGE TOTAL:

TOTAL MILEAGE TO DATE:

### INJURY

Alcohol, antihistamines, and other medications can all have a dehydrating effect. Using them just before a run can make you have to pee, compounding your risk of dehydration. Talk with your doctor about how these medications may impact your running.

### TRAINING

Learn how to breathe through the belly when you run. Here's how to practice: Lie down on your back. Keep your upper chest and shoulders still. Focus on raising your belly as you inhale. Lower your belly as you exhale. Inhale and exhale through both your nose and your mouth. You can also practice this sitting, standing, and going about the activities of your everyday life.

## NUTRITION

Protein helps repair muscles and strengthen immunity. And since protein takes longer to digest, it helps keep you fuller for longer, which can help if you're looking to shed pounds. Choose products that are lower in saturated fat, such as skinless chicken, pork, and lean cuts of beef; fish (such as salmon and tuna); soy; low-fat dairy (like yogurt and cottage cheese); and beans and lentils. It's best to get protein from whole foods, which have nutrients like fiber and iron—nutrients that engineered foods may lack.

"It's very hard in the beginning to understand that the whole idea is not to beat other runners. Eventually you learn that the biggest competition is against the little voice inside you that wants you to quit."

—DR. GEORGE SHEEHAN,
author and former columnist
for *Runner's World*

### MONDAY

Route:

Distance: Time:

NOTES:

Cross-training:

### TUESDAY

Route:

Distance: Time:

NOTES:

Cross-training:

### WEDNESDAY

Route:

Distance: Time:

NOTES:

Cross-training:

### THURSDAY

Route:

Distance: Time:

NOTES:

Cross-training:

### FRIDAY

Route:

Distance: Time:

NOTES:

Cross-training:

## SATURDAY

Route:

Distance: Time:

NOTES:

Cross-training:

## SUNDAY

Route:

Distance: Time:

NOTES:

Cross-training:

## NOTES

WEEKLY MILEAGE TOTAL:

TOTAL MILEAGE TO DATE:

### INJURY

Studies have shown that marathoners and outdoor athletes have a higher risk of skin cancers. Know what your moles look like. Look for any changes in size or color. A pimple, scratch, or bug bite should heal within a week. If it's not healing, or it's bleeding or growing, see a dermatologist. Get an annual skin cancer screening by a dermatologist, who can examine the nuances and pick up early warning signs. If you have a history of skin cancer, get checked every 6 months.

### TRAINING

Studies show logging too few hours of sleep can impair your running while compromising recovery, immunity, and mental sharpness. Because everyone requires different amounts of sleep, log your sleep time in your training journal and look for patterns specific to you. Once you figure out what works for you, shoot for that number.

## NUTRITION

Most carbs in your diet should be "slow." These are high in fiber. They're digested slowly, so they help you maintain a steady level of energy throughout a run. Fruits, whole grains, vegetables, oatmeal, and beans are all good examples of slow carbs that provide vitamins, minerals, and antioxidants to help you stay healthy and recover quickly

"Running, much like life, has its hills and valleys. On any given run, and particularly in most marathons, we come across easy stretches and seemingly impossible challenges. I have learned to just keep going. The tough moments never last, and the easy stretches are always a joy. The same is clearly true in life; if we just keep going, we'll get to that finish line with water, massages, and bananas!"

—**WILL STARR**, runner, Swarthmore, Pennsylvania, runnersworld.com/will-starr

## MONDAY

Route:

Distance: Time:

NOTES:

Cross-training:

## TUESDAY

Route:

Distance: Time:

NOTES:

Cross-training:

## WEDNESDAY

Route:

Distance: Time:

NOTES:

Cross-training:

## THURSDAY

Route:

Distance: Time:

NOTES:

Cross-training:

## FRIDAY

Route:

Distance: Time:

NOTES:

Cross-training:

## SATURDAY

Route:

Distance: Time:

NOTES:

Cross-training:

## SUNDAY

Route:

Distance: Time:

NOTES:

Cross-training:

## NOTES

WEEKLY MILEAGE TOTAL:

TOTAL MILEAGE TO DATE:

### INJURY

The health benefits of yoga have been well established: Studies have shown that yoga reduces stress, aids weight loss, and manages pain. The strength and flexibility you develop on the mat—namely in the core, quads, and hip flexors—can help you run more efficiently. But you have to shop around. There are many yoga styles and settings to choose from. No single style of yoga is best for everyone. So if on your first try you're turned off by the teacher, the atmosphere, or the poses, keep searching until you find the right fit for you.

### TRAINING

As you're looking straight ahead as you run, you shouldn't catch a glimpse of your feet in your lower peripheral vision. If you see your foot pop out in front of you, for instance, this probably means that you are overstriding or your stride rate is too low.

## JOHN MCNASBY

Loss prevention specialist
Philadelphia

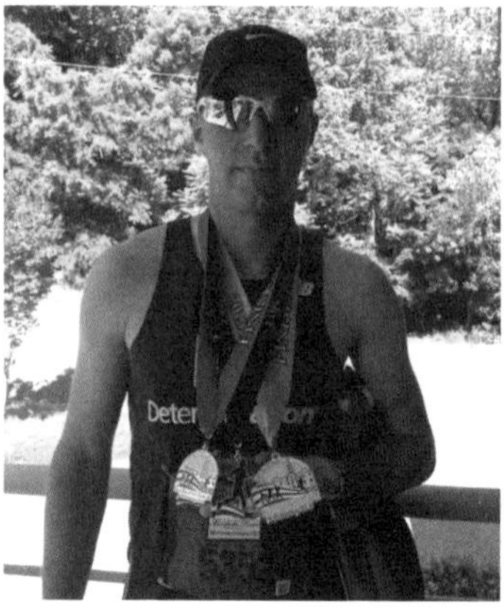


**WHAT GOT ME GOING:** After my divorce, I let myself get too heavy, and my blood pressure was horrific. I was 225 pounds and had almost 30 percent body fat and when I did a 5-K, it took me 49 minutes. Afterward, I took a good look in the mirror. I realized I had turned to alcohol and chicken wings as an answer to my problems. I decided to become a runner. Now I am 172 pounds and have less than 10 percent body fat.

**SECRET OF MY SUCCESS:** I bought running books by Dean Karnazes and Jeff Galloway and the story of Steve Prefontaine. I went to a running store and got a gait analysis and fitted for shoes. I picked a training plan and a race. Then I went to a nutritionist. I get up at 4:30 a.m. and go for a 2-mile morning jog before work as a way to wake up. Best of all, no matter what happens that day, I got a small run in. They are the slowest 2 miles I run these days. So 20 minutes and 2 miles every morning is my version of morning coffee. In terms of eating, wings, fat, liquor, candy bars, doughnuts—all that tasty stuff is gone. If I am craving a snack late at night, I'll have a piece of fruit. Now, I also cook my own food at night and bring that for lunch instead of eating fast food every day. This has kept me sane. My snacks used to be more than 300 calories; a pack of cookies, a piece of pound cake. A Hershey bar could always be found at my desk. Now my snack is a 100-calorie pack.

**HOW RUNNING CHANGED MY LIFE:** Those first few weeks, when I could hardly breathe after running for 30 seconds, I realized how out of shape I was and how much it was going to take to get to that first finish line. I got over it by realizing that I was lucky to have the chance to start over and make changes in my life. I just kept telling myself the pain and sweat would be worth it. My parents try to go to all of my races, and they look at me with such a look of pride. No matter how badly my race goes, it doesn't matter, because they are proud.

**I WISH I'D KNOWN:** Do not give up when it gets tough. It gets better. Those first few weeks may be dreadful, but you can do it. And it will be the best feeling in the world to say you are a runner.

# FOR BEGINNERS ONLY

**Q** I'm training for my first 5-K and I'm having trouble sticking to my training routine. Any suggestions for how I can stay motivated?

**A** Everyone has different reasons for running, so it's important to tap into why you began running in the first place. List your reasons for why you started training and what you hope to accomplish. That list may really provide just the motivational boost you're looking for.

When you have made your list, put it in a prominent place like the bathroom mirror or the refrigerator. After all, it's way too easy to lose focus with all the other demands of life.

Here are some other tips that may help you stick with your training:

**Pick the right training plan.** Choose a plan that fits your current level of fitness. Much like *Goldilocks and the Three Bears*, it has to be just right—not too hard and not too easy. If the plan is too hard, you risk getting injured and becoming discouraged, which can set you up for failure. On the other hand, if the plan is too easy, it will not help you get fitter. Your workouts should challenge you slightly; some moments may feel hard, but doable. You should feel a sense of accomplishment when done, not total exhaustion.

**Put your workout first.** Exercise first thing in the morning, if possible. Set out your clothes the night before, set the alarm, get up, and go before you even have time to think about it. When we plan to work out at the end of the day, we have all day to talk ourselves out of it! Fatigue, family, or work commitments can often interfere with even the best of intentions. Getting a run in first thing in the morning will help you start the day with a feeling of accomplishment.

**Set small goals.** Break your 5-K goal down into smaller segments. Focus on running for short time intervals or short distances like a 1/4 mile first, rather than the entire 3.1 miles. Increase the distance or time you run in small segments. Look ahead to sign up for future races to help keep you training. Target something that interests you or challenges you—like a trail race, a longer distance, or a destination race to keep your running life exciting!

**Keep track.** Measure your resting heart rate, blood pressure, weight, percent body fat, and/or waist and hip measurements to help track your transformation along with tracking your mileage. Seeing the results of all your hard work on the road can help keep you on track. Your resting heart rate and blood pressure should become lower as your fitness level improves. In this training journal, keep track of how all these factors change over time. And take notes on how your quality of life is changing. How do your clothes fit? How do you feel? Do you have more energy throughout the day? Are you sleeping better? Even the subtlest changes can help keep you on track.

*Coach and exercise physiologist Susan Paul, author of "For Beginners Only" column,* Runner's World, *is program manager for the Track Shack Foundation. Paul has coached is program director for the Orlando Track Shack Foundation. For more information, visit trackshack.com.*

WEEK 43 WEEK OF TO

## NUTRITION

Seafood is an excellent source of hard-to-come-by omega-3 fatty acids, which promote heart health and fight inflammation. Fish and seafood are also an excellent source of protein and many vitamins and minerals. Consume seafood at least once a week. Choose fish such as anchovies, flounder, salmon, sole, shrimp, scallops, clams, and oysters. Worried about mercury? Avoid larger fish like marlin, swordfish, and shark.

"The greatest pleasure in life is doing the things people say we cannot do."

—**WALTER BAGEHOT,** British journalist and economist

### MONDAY

Route:

Distance: Time:

NOTES:

Cross-training:

### TUESDAY

Route:

Distance: Time:

NOTES:

Cross-training:

### WEDNESDAY

Route:

Distance: Time:

NOTES:

Cross-training:

### THURSDAY

Route:

Distance: Time:

NOTES:

Cross-training:

### FRIDAY

Route:

Distance: Time:

NOTES:

Cross-training:

## SATURDAY

Route:

Distance: Time:

NOTES:

Cross-training:

## SUNDAY

Route:

Distance: Time:

NOTES:

Cross-training:

## NOTES

WEEKLY MILEAGE TOTAL:

TOTAL MILEAGE TO DATE:

## INJURY

Strength training will decrease your risk of injury and help you run more efficiently. That said, you've got to bring the same dedication that you bring to your running. If you don't push yourself, you're not going to get stronger. Start with three or four times a week. Start with weights you can lift for 15 reps and build up to doing three sets of 20 to 30 repetitions. You must maintain good form throughout the movement.

## TRAINING

Your body is going to adapt to any given strength training routine in about 4 to 6 weeks. To avoid hitting a plateau and getting frustrated, add more weights, more reps, or do different exercises to target your muscle groups.

WEEK 44 WEEK OF TO

## NUTRITION

Even if it's labeled 100 percent juice, it's best to avoid juice altogether. It does contain vitamins and minerals, but juice is full of calories and sugar and devoid of fiber that will fill you up and keep you satisfied. It's harder for the body to register "I'm full" when you drink your calories.

"Do a little more each day than you think you possibly can."

—**LOWELL THOMAS**, poet

### MONDAY

Route:

Distance: Time:

NOTES:

Cross-training:

### TUESDAY

Route:

Distance: Time:

NOTES:

Cross-training:

### WEDNESDAY

Route:

Distance: Time:

NOTES:

Cross-training:

### THURSDAY

Route:

Distance: Time:

NOTES:

Cross-training:

### FRIDAY

Route:

Distance: Time:

NOTES:

Cross-training:

## SATURDAY

Route:

Distance: Time:

NOTES:

Cross-training:

## SUNDAY

Route:

Distance: Time:

NOTES:

Cross-training:

## NOTES

WEEKLY MILEAGE TOTAL:

TOTAL MILEAGE TO DATE:

### INJURY

Though many people cross-train to prevent injuries, it is possible to hurt yourself in the process. If you're injured, ask your doctor which activities are safe before you hit the gym. And before you try any machine for the first time, ask someone who works at the gym to show you how to use it and to watch you and help you maintain proper form.

### TRAINING

Training seldom goes exactly according to plan. Work or family obligations come up; illness or injury derails your runs. In general, if you miss a week of training, you can jump back into your plan as long as you were consistent for at least 4 to 6 weeks before your break. But if your downtime stretches any longer, come back more slowly. Don't try to cram in the runs you've missed. This may increase your risk of injury.

# WEEK 45 WEEK OF ____ TO ____

## NUTRITION

Avoid butter and lard and margarines that contain trans fats. They are linked to increased risk of obesity and heart disease. Instead, choose oils (like canola, olive, and grapeseed). What to spread on your toast? Choose a vegetable-oil-based spread like Promise, which contains significantly less saturated fat and is almost always cholesterol free.

"If you run, you are a runner. It doesn't matter how fast or how far. It doesn't matter if today is your first day or if you've been running for 20 years. There is no test to pass, no license to earn, no membership card to get. You just run."

—**JOHN BINGHAM,** running speaker and writer

## MONDAY

Route:

Distance: Time:

NOTES:

Cross-training:

## TUESDAY

Route:

Distance: Time:

NOTES:

Cross-training:

## WEDNESDAY

Route:

Distance: Time:

NOTES:

Cross-training:

## THURSDAY

Route:

Distance: Time:

NOTES:

Cross-training:

## FRIDAY

Route:

Distance: Time:

NOTES:

Cross-training:

## SATURDAY

Route:

Distance: Time:

NOTES:

Cross-training:

## SUNDAY

Route:

Distance: Time:

NOTES:

Cross-training:

## NOTES

WEEKLY MILEAGE TOTAL:

TOTAL MILEAGE TO DATE:

### INJURY

Whenever you do any new strength-training routine, you're bound to be sore for 1 to 2 days afterward. You shouldn't be so sore that you can't go about your daily activities, but you should feel a general muscle achiness. But after a few weeks of doing that same routine, the soreness will go away.

### TRAINING

In the winter, look for snow that's been packed down—it will provide better traction. Fresh powder can cover up ice patches. Run on the street if it's been plowed, provided that it's safe from traffic, and watch out for areas that could have black ice. Use the sidewalk if it's clear of ice and slippery snow. Find a well-lit route, slow your pace, and make sure you're familiar with areas of broken concrete.

WEEK **46** WEEK OF ____ TO ____

## NUTRITION

Nuts come packed with fiber, protein, vitamins, minerals, and antioxidants and have been linked to lower risk of heart disease. Avoid nuts that are roasted or coated in oil and that have other added sugars and fillers. Avoid highly processed nut butters with a laundry list of preservatives and fillers like sugar, soy lecithin, and hydrogenated vegetable oils. Look for raw, ground, or dry-roasted nuts that are free of fillers and preservatives.

"Running is easy: Put one foot in front of the other. Staying motivated to run requires much more. It takes thinking and planning. It takes believing in yourself and the value of your workout time. It takes a powerful web of attitudes and practices that make your daily exercise as regular as, you know, brushing your teeth."

—**AMBY BURFOOT**, 1968 Boston Marathon winner, *Runner's World* editor at large

## MONDAY

Route:

Distance: Time:

NOTES:

Cross-training:

## TUESDAY

Route:

Distance: Time:

NOTES:

Cross-training:

## WEDNESDAY

Route:

Distance: Time:

NOTES:

Cross-training:

## THURSDAY

Route:

Distance: Time:

NOTES:

Cross-training:

## FRIDAY

Route:

Distance: Time:

NOTES:

Cross-training:

## SATURDAY

Route:

Distance: Time:

NOTES:

Cross-training:

## SUNDAY

Route:

Distance: Time:

NOTES:

Cross-training:

## NOTES

WEEKLY MILEAGE TOTAL:

TOTAL MILEAGE TO DATE:

### INJURY

With basic strength-training exercises, go slow. If you're just whipping through it to get it over with, and not focusing on form, you're not going to get the benefits. Plus, if you're not doing it with the right form, you're setting yourself up for injury. To slow down, count out "one, two" as you lift the weight, holding it for one count, then counting out "one, two" as you release the weight.

### TRAINING

In order to build your overall fitness on a treadmill, it's a good idea to do faster workouts with no incline as well as slower-paced workouts with an incline. The uphill workouts build strength, while the faster flat workouts help you develop stamina, endurance, and quick footwork. Adjust both speed and incline during your workout, and you can better simulate the changing terrain of a road run.

WEEK 47 WEEK OF ______ TO ______

## NUTRITION

If you're peeling or removing the rind (avocado, bananas, or onions), conventionally grown produce is fine. If you're going to eat the exterior (apples, peaches, bell peppers), buying organic will limit your exposure to pesticides and other substances.

"Even when you have gone as far as you can, and everything hurts, and you are staring at the specter of self-doubt, you can find a bit more strength deep inside you, if you look closely enough."

—**HAL HIGDON**, coach and author

### MONDAY

**Route:**

**Distance:** **Time:**

**NOTES:**

**Cross-training:**

### TUESDAY

**Route:**

**Distance:** **Time:**

**NOTES:**

**Cross-training:**

### WEDNESDAY

**Route:**

**Distance:** **Time:**

**NOTES:**

**Cross-training:**

### THURSDAY

**Route:**

**Distance:** **Time:**

**NOTES:**

**Cross-training:**

### FRIDAY

**Route:**

**Distance:** **Time:**

**NOTES:**

**Cross-training:**

## SATURDAY

Route:

Distance: Time:

NOTES:

Cross-training:

## SUNDAY

Route:

Distance: Time:

NOTES:

Cross-training:

## NOTES

WEEKLY MILEAGE TOTAL:

TOTAL MILEAGE TO DATE:

### INJURY

Damp clothing increases heat loss. Immediately after your workout, remove your sweaty clothes and get into a hot shower—or, if you aren't ready for a shower yet, into something dry and cozy.

### TRAINING

When it's windy outside, if you can, start your walk or run facing the wind and finish with it at your back. Otherwise, you'll work up a sweat and then turn directly into a cold blast. You can break this into segments, walking or running into the wind for 10 minutes, turning around to walk or run with the wind at your back for 5 minutes, and repeating.

WEEK **48** WEEK OF TO

## NUTRITION

Frozen meals are convenient and the portions are measured out for you, but they can be filled with calories, fat, and sodium. Avoid any product with more than 500 calories, 10 grams of fat, or more than 500 grams of sodium per serving. And check the serving size before you dig in. Lots of meals that look like they're a single serving are actually two.

"Running is the greatest metaphor for life, because you get out of it what you put into it."

—OPRAH WINFREY, talk show host

### MONDAY

Route:

Distance: Time:

NOTES:

Cross-training:

### TUESDAY

Route:

Distance: Time:

NOTES:

Cross-training:

### WEDNESDAY

Route:

Distance: Time:

NOTES:

Cross-training:

### THURSDAY

Route:

Distance: Time:

NOTES:

Cross-training:

### FRIDAY

Route:

Distance: Time:

NOTES:

Cross-training:

## SATURDAY

Route:

Distance: Time:

NOTES:

Cross-training:

## SUNDAY

Route:

Distance: Time:

NOTES:

Cross-training:

## NOTES

WEEKLY MILEAGE TOTAL:

TOTAL MILEAGE TO DATE:

### INJURY

Cover your extremities when it's cold outside. Your nose, fingers, and ears are the first to freeze, so be sure to keep them well protected from wind, wet, and freezing temperatures. Balaclavas—knit masks that cover the whole head, with holes for nose and eyes—are the way to go. Or try a heavy synthetic knit cap pulled down low, with a scarf or neck muffler pulled up high.

### TRAINING

The term *split* refers to the time it takes to complete any defined distance. If you're running 1 mile, or four laps around the track, you might check your split after you have covered four laps.

## CHRISTINE C. CASADY

University IT
East Norriton, Pennsylvania

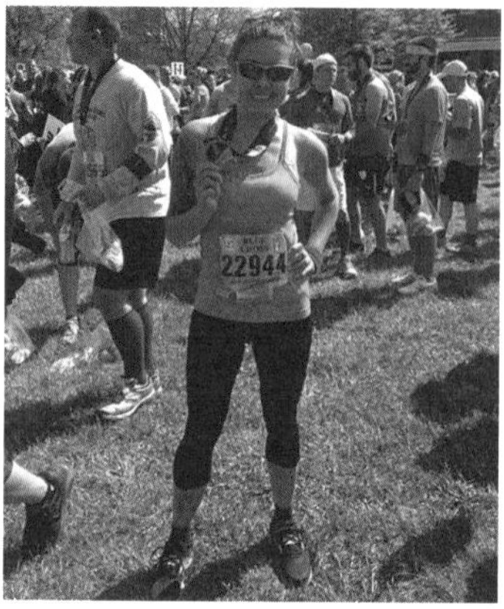


**WHAT GOT ME GOING:** For about 2 years I was dealing with my physical and emotional battle with infertility issues. In March of 2012 I had reached a point where I had done all I could up to that moment and I was able to put all my medical issues up on a shelf for a bit. Having been focused on that for so long, I found myself feeling like I needed to start a new chapter in my life. I needed something to help pull me out of my hole that I had been in for so long.

**SECRET OF MY SUCCESS:** I started by trying classes at a new gym. It took place outdoors at a local park every week. It involved 4 miles of running on trails and pavements and included intervals and sprints. I had never run anything like this, or with a group.

**HOW RUNNING CHANGED MY LIFE:** It turned out to be the turning point in my life. I drew strength from the encouragement and camaraderie I got from others; I found happiness completing the running class successfully, and I felt invigorated by the intensity of the workout. When the class was over, I was glowing and never looked back! It was a stepping-stone for future increased miles, races, relationships, and friendships. I found hope, love, recovery, and life in running. In so many ways, it changed my life forever. I have built friendships that have become the center of my happiness. I have a confidence in myself that I've lacked most of my life. And through the ups and downs of running, I have found new perspective in life. The suffering and success has made me a stronger, happier person. I'll never look back.

**I WISH I'D KNOWN:** Don't let fear ever stop you from moving forward. Put one foot in front of the other and move. Before you know it, you will be accomplishing distances and speeds you never thought possible.

# FOR BEGINNERS ONLY

**Q** Should I join a running group?

**A** Running tends to be a solo sport, and we tend to be creatures of habit, running the same routes, at the same time, at the same pace, day in and day out. Although that can help keep us consistent, it can also contribute to burnout, boredom, and a feeling of staleness over time. Joining up with a group can be a great change of pace, even when that group's routine is different than our own. The social interaction, especially on a long run, can be invaluable! Conversation offers a great distraction and helps the miles fly by, and a group can help you discover new routes in your area that you can later take on when you go solo.

To find a running group near you, check your local specialty running shop, forums like the ones on runnersworld.com, or find one at rrca.org. Many running groups have organized training programs in the spring and fall. Before joining up with the group for the first time, it's a good idea to contact the group leader to find out about the route, the usual pace of the run, distance the group is running, and if any of the runners use walk breaks. Also, you may want to find out if the group supplies water or whether you should carry your own. As much as possible, get a feel for the general experience level of the group. Is it full of runners of all abilities—and is it likely you'll find someone to run with who is at your level of fitness?

When you're on the run, be sure to follow some basic group etiquette. Give others enough space by not crowding too close to them. And if you're in front of others, point out any obstacles like holes, debris, puddles, or oncoming cyclists and traffic.

It's OK to mix up your training and do some runs with others on your own. Many runners do their usual training during the week and then on some weekends. For longer runs, you can opt to join the group for some social time. As runners, we tend to savor routine and become very set in our ways, so using different run routes, running at different times of the day, running continuously, and also running with walk breaks is a great way to keep your running routine fresh and prevent burnout. After all, variety is the spice of life!

*Coach and exercise physiologist Susan Paul, author of "For Beginners Only" column,* Runner's World, *is program manager for the Track Shack Foundation. Paul has coached is program director for the Orlando Track Shack Foundation. For more information, visit trackshack.com.*

WEEK **49** WEEK OF TO

## NUTRITION

Looking for the perfect pasta? Choose whole wheat, brown rice, buckwheat, spelt, or other varieties with at least 5 grams of fiber per 2-ounce serving. It should also have at least 6 grams of protein. And what about the sauce? Make sure it has less than 400 milligrams of sodium, less than 4 grams of sugar, and 2 grams of fat or less per half-cup serving.

"Remember, the feeling you get from a good run is far better than the feeling you get from sitting around wishing you were running."

—**SARAH CONDOR**, runner and author

## MONDAY

Route:

Distance: Time:

NOTES:

Cross-training:

## TUESDAY

Route:

Distance: Time:

NOTES:

Cross-training:

## WEDNESDAY

Route:

Distance: Time:

NOTES:

Cross-training:

## THURSDAY

Route:

Distance: Time:

NOTES:

Cross-training:

## FRIDAY

Route:

Distance: Time:

NOTES:

Cross-training:

## SATURDAY

**Route:**

**Distance:** **Time:**

**NOTES:**

**Cross-training:**

## SUNDAY

**Route:**

**Distance:** **Time:**

**NOTES:**

**Cross-training:**

## NOTES

## WEEKLY MILEAGE TOTAL:

## TOTAL MILEAGE TO DATE:

## INJURY

As long as you're dressed for the conditions, you can produce enough body heat to offset the cold. Still, when it is cold outside, watch out for hypothermia and frostbite. Hypothermia strikes when your body loses more heat than it can produce. Symptoms can start with shivering and numbness and progress to lack of coordination. You're most at risk when it's rainy or snowy and your skin is damp. Frostbite most commonly strikes the nose, ears, cheeks, fingers, and toes. It can start with tingling, burning, aching, and redness, then progress to numbness. Windy and wet days are the riskiest times for frostbite.

## TRAINING

Create space between your shoulders and your ears when you run. It's common to tense up the shoulders, especially when you feel fatigued. But that uses extra energy your legs and lungs need to run strong.

## NUTRITION

Whole milk, cheese, and yogurt are packed with sugar and fat that you don't need. When looking for milk, choose fat-free or 1% versions, or try other nondairy milks like almond and soy milk. Try low-fat cheeses and sour cream. With yogurt, choose brands with less than 5 grams of sugar per serving. Or better yet, buy plain Greek yogurt and sweeten it by adding your own fresh fruit.

"Don't bother just to be better than your contemporaries or predecessors. Try to be better than yourself."

—WILLIAM FAULKNER, author

### MONDAY

Route:

Distance: Time:

NOTES:

Cross-training:

### TUESDAY

Route:

Distance: Time:

NOTES:

Cross-training:

### WEDNESDAY

Route:

Distance: Time:

NOTES:

Cross-training:

### THURSDAY

Route:

Distance: Time:

NOTES:

Cross-training:

### FRIDAY

Route:

Distance: Time:

NOTES:

Cross-training:

## SATURDAY

Route:

Distance: Time:

NOTES:

Cross-training:

## SUNDAY

Route:

Distance: Time:

NOTES:

Cross-training:

## NOTES

WEEKLY MILEAGE TOTAL:

TOTAL MILEAGE TO DATE:

## INJURY

Make sure your arms are moving straight forward and back when you run, and not crossing your body. Think about running with your thumbs up to prevent crossing over your midline. Your elbows should be popping back, not trying to punch forward.

## TRAINING

While there's nothing as convenient as stepping out your front door and going around the block, if that's not safe you have other options. Treadmills offer a cushioned, more forgiving alternative to pavement, and they allow you to get your workout in all weather conditions. Tracks are ideal places to take your first steps, since they're flat, traffic free, and the distance is measured. Most tracks are 400 meters around, so four laps is roughly equivalent to 1 mile.

WEEK 51 WEEK OF ______ TO ______

## NUTRITION

Don't grocery shop when you're hungry! This can prompt you to make unhealthy choices. Eat before you leave home.

"A few people will never miss a chance to tear down running. The best response is to continue running and loving it."

—**Mark Remy**, author and *Runner's World* editor at large

### MONDAY

Route:

Distance: Time:

NOTES:

Cross-training:

### TUESDAY

Route:

Distance: Time:

NOTES:

Cross-training:

### WEDNESDAY

Route:

Distance: Time:

NOTES:

Cross-training:

### THURSDAY

Route:

Distance: Time:

NOTES:

Cross-training:

### FRIDAY

Route:

Distance: Time:

NOTES:

Cross-training:

## SATURDAY

Route:

Distance: Time:

NOTES:

Cross-training:

## SUNDAY

Route:

Distance: Time:

NOTES:

Cross-training:

## NOTES

WEEKLY MILEAGE TOTAL:

TOTAL MILEAGE TO DATE:

### INJURY

As sore as you might feel the day after a race, the next day, get going. It's important to do some sort of nonimpact activity like swimming, cycling, or working out on the elliptical trainer. The movement will increase circulation to your sore muscles and help you bounce back sooner. Just keep the effort level easy.

### TRAINING

Many runners find that races jump-start a routine that's become a rut. When you put a race on your calendar, you'll find more motivation for logging those miles.

WEEK 52 WEEK OF TO

## NUTRITION

The 30 to 60 minutes after your workout is prime time for recovery. That's when your body is superprimed to restock glycogen stores and start repairing muscle tissue so you can bounce back for your next workout. Make sure to have a healthy meal with a carbs-to-protein ratio of 2:1.

"Even a bad run is better than none at all."

—SUZANNE PERRAULT, *Runner's World* managing editor

### MONDAY

Route:

Distance: Time:

NOTES:

Cross-training:

### TUESDAY

Route:

Distance: Time:

NOTES:

Cross-training:

### WEDNESDAY

Route:

Distance: Time:

NOTES:

Cross-training:

### THURSDAY

Route:

Distance: Time:

NOTES:

Cross-training:

### FRIDAY

Route:

Distance: Time:

NOTES:

Cross-training:

## SATURDAY

Route:

Distance: Time:

NOTES:

Cross-training:

## SUNDAY

Route:

Distance: Time:

NOTES:

Cross-training:

## NOTES

WEEKLY MILEAGE TOTAL:

TOTAL MILEAGE TO DATE:

## INJURY

Find a health-care provider who has experience treating athletes and keeping them on the road. Doctors with added training in sports medicine are often the best place to start, especially for a new problem. Sports docs can give you a comprehensive evaluation that includes diagnostic tests, from blood counts to bone scans to MRIs. They may refer you to a specialist to rehab injuries.

## TRAINING

Racing? Set one goal for a perfect race and another as a backup in case it's hot, it's windy, or it's just not your day. If something makes your first goal impossible halfway through, you'll need another goal to motivate you to finish strong. And it's best to set a third goal that has nothing to do with your finishing time. This goal could be something like finishing, or running up the hills rather than walking them.

# YOUR FIRST (START WALKING) TRAINING PLAN

*Runner's World*'s Start Walking plan, designed by coach and exercise physiologist Janet Hamilton, owner of Atlanta-based RunningStrong.com, will help you get in the habit of regular exercise and lay the foundation for your running life. With this 7-week plan, you can build up to 150 minutes per week—about 30 minutes five times a week—the amount that the American College of Sports Medicine says will stave off diabetes, heart disease, and stroke; lower blood pressure and cholesterol; increase energy; and improve depression and anxiety. These walks should be brisk. You can substitute time on a stationary bike or an elliptical trainer, but walking is the best foundation for running. If you don't have time for the longest workout of each week, it's okay to split it in half. You'll get the same health benefits. If you have a BMI of at least 25, are 60 or older, or if you'd like to take a more gradual approach, you can repeat any week, or every week, and stretch this out to an 8-, 10-, or 12-week plan.

| | MONDAY | TUESDAY | WEDNESDAY | THURSDAY |
|---|---|---|---|---|
| **Week 1** | 15 min | 25 min | Rest or optional 15 min walk | 25 min |
| **Week 2** | 15 min | 28 min | Rest or optional 15 min walk | 28 min |
| **Week 3** | 20 min | 30 min | Rest or optional 15 min walk | 30 min |
| **Week 4** | 20 min | 35 min | Rest or optional 15 min walk | 35 min |
| **Week 5** | 20 min | 40 min | Rest or optional 20 min walk | 40 min |
| **Week 6** | 20 min | 40 min | Rest or optional 20 min walk | 40 min |
| **Week 7** | 20 min | 45 min | Rest or optional 20 min walk | 40 min |

| | FRIDAY | SATURDAY | SUNDAY | TOTAL MINUTES (estimated mileage) |
|---|---|---|---|---|
| | Rest | 35 min | Rest | 100–115 min (5–7.7 mi.) |
| | Rest | 38 min | Rest | 109–124 min (5.4–8.3 mi) |
| | Rest | 40 min | Rest | 120–135 min (6–9 mi) |
| | Rest | 45 min | Rest | 135–150 min (6.7–10 mi) |
| | Rest | 50 min | Rest | 150–170 min (7.5–11.3 mi) |
| | Rest | 55 min | Rest | 155–175 min (7.8–11.7 mi) |
| | Rest | 60 min | Rest | 165–185 min (8.25–12.3 mi) |

# TIPS FOR YOUR FIRST RACE

Even for seasoned runners, the days before a race can be stressful. With all the hope and hard work that you invested in your goal event, you want to arrive at the starting line feeling calm, healthy, and ready to do your best. These tips will keep you on track in the critical days and hours before the starting gun fires and will help you recover after you cross the finish line.

## The Days Before the Race

**DON'T DO ANYTHING NEW.** This isn't the time to try new shoes, food or drinks, gear, or anything else you haven't used on several training runs. Stick with the routine that works for you.

**GRAZE, DON'T CHOW DOWN.** Rather than devouring a gigantic bowl of pasta the night before the race, which could upset your stomach, try eating carbs in small increments throughout the day before the race.

**REVIEW THIS LOG.** If you're feeling nervous, go back and add up all the mileage you've done. Draw confidence from everything you've already accomplished, from how many days you got out the door when you would have preferred to sleep in. Approach the race as a victory lap and a celebration of all the hard work that you did to get to the starting line.

## Race Day

**DON'T OVERDRESS.** It will probably be cool at the start, but don't wear more clothing than you need. To stay warm at the start, bring clothes that you can throw off after the first few miles.

**FIRST TIME? JUST FOCUS ON FINISHING.** Anytime you are completing a race distance for the first time, you should forget about time goals and focus on finishing feeling strong, happy, and ready to race again. After your body learns what it takes to go that distance, you can start thinking about finishing faster.

**IF IT'S NOT YOUR FIRST TIME, SET MULTIPLE GOALS.** Set one goal for a perfect race and another as a backup in case it's hot, windy, or just not your day. If something makes your first goal impossible halfway through the race, you'll need another goal to motivate you to finish strong.

**FIX IT SOONER, NOT LATER.** Early in the race, if your shoelace becomes untied or you start to chafe, take care of it before it becomes really painful later in the race.
**LINE UP EARLY.** You don't want to be rushing to the starting line, so don't wait for the last call to get there.
**START SLOW AND STAY EVEN.** When the starting gun fires, everyone will take off like they're being chased. Don't follow them. If you start out too fast, you risk burning out early and struggling to finish. Start slow with the idea that you're going to finish feeling strong. This can take a lot of discipline; it's mentally tough to have so many people pass you, and you may be convinced that you'll be the last person to finish the race. But there's a good chance you won't be. In fact you'll probably pass a lot of those people late in the race.

## After the Race

**KEEP MOVING.** Cross the finish line and keep walking for a few minutes to fend off stiffness and gradually bring your heart rate back to its resting state.
**REFUEL.** Within 30 minutes of finishing, refuel with healthy carbs and sources of lean protein. If you can't eat postrace, pack a recovery drink in your gear bag. Within a few hours try to eat a regular healthy meal with carbs and protein.
**GET WARM.** Change out of the clothes you ran in and get into dry clothes as soon as possible. After you cross the finish line, your core temperature will start to drop, and keeping sweaty clothes on will keep you cold.
**THE NEXT DAY, GET GOING.** As sore as you might feel the day after the race, it's important to do some sort of nonimpact activity like swimming, cycling, or working out on the elliptical trainer. The movement will increase circulation to your sore muscles and help you bounce back sooner. Just keep the effort level easy.

# HOW FAST CAN YOU FINISH?

This chart helps you calculate your average pace for these popular race distances. Find your time per mile in the column on the left and find the equivalent race finish time.

| PACE [average time/mile] | 5-K FINISH TIME | 10-K FINISH TIME | HALF-MARATHON FINISH TIME | MARATHON FINISH TIME |
|---|---|---|---|---|
| 3:00 | 40:18 | 1:20:36 | 2:50:15 | 5:40:35 |
| 12:30 | 38:45 | 1:17:30 | 2:43:45 | 5:27:30 |
| 12:00 | 37:12 | 1:14:24 | 2:37:11 | 5:14:23 |
| 11:30 | 35:38 | 1:11:17 | 2:30:39 | 5:01:18 |
| 11:00 | 34:06 | 1:08:12 | 2:24:05 | 4:48:11 |
| 10:30 | 32:33 | 1:05:06 | 2:17:32 | 4:35:05 |
| 10:00 | 31:00 | 1:02:00 | 2:11:00 | 4:22:00 |
| 9:45 | 30:13 | 1:00:27 | 2:07:43 | 4:15:26 |
| 9:30 | 29:26 | 58:53 | 2:04:27 | 4:08:54 |
| 9:00 | 27:54 | 55:48 | 1:57:53 | 3:55:47 |
| 8:45 | 27:07 | 54:15 | 1:54:37 | 3:49:15 |
| 8:30 | 26:21 | 52:42 | 1:51:20 | 3:42:41 |
| 8:15 | 25:34 | 51:08 | 1:48:04 | 3:36:09 |
| 8:00 | 24:48 | 49:36 | 1:44:47 | 3:29:35 |
| 7:45 | 24:01 | 48:03 | 1:41:31 | 3:23:02 |
| 7:30 | 23:15 | 46:30 | 1:38:15 | 3:16:30 |

# A GUIDE TO COMMON RUNNING TERMS

## A

**ACHILLES TENDON:** The tendon along the back of your foot that attaches your calf muscles to your heel bone. Achilles tendinitis can occur in new runners who increase their distance and/or intensity too quickly. This is especially true of new runners who have been inactive in recent years and who often wear heeled shoes (which can make the Achilles tendon shorter and tighter). Good flexibility in your calves and ankles can help to take some of the load off the Achilles tendon.

**AID STATION:** Also called a water stop. Any point along the course that offers water and sports drinks, handed out by volunteers. Often at bigger races people also hand out gels, energy bars, and other items.

**ALTITUDE TRAINING:** Elite runners train at altitude to increase their number of red blood cells, improving oxygen delivery to their muscles. At altitude, the amount of oxygen in the blood is reduced because there's less oxygen in the air. The kidneys then secrete more of a hormone called erythropoietin (EPO), which causes the body to create more red blood cells. Runners find they can train harder and perform better for several weeks after they return from about a monthlong stay at altitude. If that's not possible, arriving at altitude just 24 hours before the start is your best bet. You won't acclimate, but you'll limit your exposure to some of the negative effects of the thin air, such as dehydration and disturbed sleep. Start your race slower and build intensity. Expect race times to be slower. Dehydration can occur at altitude because the air is thinner and drier, so drink plenty of fluids. Get plenty of rest and allow a few weeks back at lower altitudes before you race again.

**AQUA JOGGING:** Running against the water's resistance in the deep end, where you can't touch the bottom, provides many of the benefits of running on land. A flotation belt will help keep you upright and give you stability.

**ATHENA:** Races will often have divisions designated as "Athena" or "filly" for female runners who are over a certain weight. The minimum weight to qualify for that division varies from race to race.

## B

**BANDIT:** Someone who is participating in the race unofficially, without having registered or paid for an entry.

**BIB:** The sheets printed with numbers (called "bib numbers") used to identify each runner in a race.

**BLACK TOENAILS:** Lots of downhill running and too-small shoes can cause these, because both situations cause your toes to slam into the front of your shoe. They typically heal on their own within a few months.

**BLOODY NIPPLES:** These are often caused by chafing, friction caused by the rubbing of the nipples against the shirt while running. They're more common in men and during cold weather, and they can be remedied by covering your nipples with adhesive bandages or nipple guards, which are sold in many specialty running stores.

**BODY MASS INDEX (BMI):** A simple estimation of body fat that can be used to determine whether or not your weight is healthy. BMI is derived by comparing your height to your weight. It can be used by men and women of all ages.

**BQ:** Shorthand for Boston Qualifying time. Often used to describe a marathon or half-marathon finish time that qualifies a person for entry into the Boston Marathon.

**BRICK WORKOUT:** A workout that includes consecutive biking and running. Often used by triathletes and duathletes to prepare for their goal events.

## C

**CARB-LOADING:** The practice of increasing the percentage of carbs in your diet during the days leading up to an endurance event such as a marathon, half-marathon, or even a long training run. (Note: Carb-loading is not simply eating more of everything.) Carb-loading stores glycogen in the muscles and liver so that it can be used during the race; it is most effective when done along with a taper. Make sure your food choices are carbohydrate rich, not full of fat. For example, choose spaghetti with red sauce instead of Alfredo sauce, or a bagel instead of a croissant.

**CERTIFIED COURSE:** Most marathons and half-marathons, and many 5-Ks and 10-Ks, are certified by USA Track & Field, which ensures that the distance of the race is accurately measured. For any running performance to be accepted as a record or for national ranking, it has to be run on a USATF-certified course.

**CHAFING:** Bloodied, blistered skin caused by friction that happens after clothing-on-skin or skin-on-skin rubbing.

**CHIP:** A small plastic piece attached to a runner's shoelace that's used to track a runner's progress and record times during a race. Timing chips are activated once you step over the electronic mat at the start and finish of a race, and at various points in between. At most races, if you forget your timing chip, your race time will not be officially recorded.

**CLYDESDALE:** Races often have divisions designated as "Clydesdale" for male runners who are over a certain weight. The minimum weight to qualify for that division varies from race to race.

**COOLDOWN:** A period of light physical activity, like walking, after a longer or harder run. Done to help bring the heart rate down gradually and prevent the blood from pooling in the legs.

**CORRAL:** A sectioned area at the lineup of a race that helps separate athletes into different pace groups. The faster an individual is, the more likely he or she will end up in one of the first few corrals. These corrals are especially important at large races, such as marathons, where elite athletes are running.

## E

**ENDORPHINS:** Brain chemicals long credited with producing a "runner's high," the sense of elation that runners report experiencing. More recent research attributes this to endocannabinoids, molecules created by the body that are said to reduce pain and anxiety and promote well-being.

## F

**FARTLEK:** Speed play, or *fartlek* in Swedish (the concept originated in Sweden), is a speedwork format in which you run faster for however long (or short) you want.

**5-K:** A race that's 3.1 miles long. It's the most popular race distance in the United States, and a good distance for your first race.

## G

**GLYCOGEN:** The form of carbohydrates that is stored in your muscles and liver and is converted to glucose for energy during exercise. The amount of stored glycogen depends on your level of training and the amount of carbohydrates in your diet. The glycogen that is stored (so it can be made available for use during a race) increases during periods of carb-loading.

**GPS:** Many running watches now have a GPS function that tracks your distance with a fairly high degree of accuracy. This can be helpful when you're running new routes. But always remember that a GPS unit is a tool that might help your running rather than something you have to answer to. There's no inherent magic in standard measures of distance like a mile or kilometer. So don't feel obligated to keep running until your GPS says you've run exactly a given distance. Most experienced runners learn to estimate their run lengths and figure their mileage averages out to near accuracy over time.

## H

**HALF-MARATHON:** A race that's 13.1 miles long. The half-marathon has been the fastest-growing race distance in the United States in the last few years. Many runners like the challenge of extending their endurance without having to do the training necessary to finish a marathon.

**HAMSTRINGS:** The long muscles along the back of your legs. Strong, supple hamstrings are crucial for running your best, because they help to flex your knees and extend your hips. Weak or tight hamstrings shift some of the work of running to other body parts that aren't as well equipped for the job. New runners whose daily lives involve a lot of sitting should include hamstring-strengthening and flexibility exercises in their routine from the start.

**HEART RATE:** The number of times your heart beats in a minute. Training by heart rate accounts for many variables that affect how you feel from day to day. This makes it a better way to monitor how hard you're working than an arbitrary measure such as your pace. The key is to know what your maximum heart rate is; once you know that, you can figure out the range of heart rates that correspond to the effort level you want for a given run.

**HEAT INDEX:** A combined measurement of temperature and humidity that shows how hot it feels outside. When humidity is high, it cripples the body's ability to sweat—the body's self-cooling mechanism—so the body retains more heat and it's riskier to be outside. High humidity also increases the risk for conditions like heat cramps, heat exhaustion, and heatstroke. The National Weather Service issues an alert when the heat index is expected to exceed 105° to 110°F for at least 2 consecutive days.

**HILL REPEATS:** A workout that includes sprinting uphill fast, jogging downhill at an easy pace to recover, and then repeating the sequence. It's thought to be an efficient way to build leg strength, speed, and aerobic capacity. Hill repeats reduce your injury risk because they limit fast-running time and because the incline of a hill shortens the distance your feet have to fall, reducing the impact of each step.

## I

**ICE BATH:** Typically taken after long runs, races, and hard workouts, ice baths involve immersing your legs in ice water for 15 to 20 minutes. The ice constricts blood vessels and decreases metabolic activity, which reduces swelling and tissue breakdown. Once you get out of the cold water, the underlying tissues warm up, causing a return of faster blood flow, which helps flush waste products out of the cells.

**ILIOTIBIAL BAND:** A thick, fibrous band that connects your hips and knees. It helps to flex and rotate your hips and stabilize and extend your knees. It can easily become strained, leading to iliotibial (IT) band syndrome, if you increase your mileage too quickly. The IT band is also often irritated on the leg farther away from traffic if you regularly run on canted roads.

**INTERVAL TRAINING:** Technically, this refers to the time you spend recovering between speed segments. But the term is commonly used to refer to track workouts in general or fast bouts of running.

## L

**LONG SLOW DISTANCE (LSD) RUNS:** Any run that's longer than a weekly run, which is the foundation of marathon and half-marathon training. These workouts help build endurance and psychological toughness that can help you get through race day.

## M

**MARATHON:** A race that's 26.2 miles long. Although many runners are understandably proud of having run a marathon, some of the greatest runners in history have never done one, so don't feel like you have to do a marathon to call yourself a runner. Most experts agree that you should have a year of regular running under your belt before you start training for your first marathon.

**MINIMALISM:** A recent movement in running shoes away from the highly cushioned, thickly heeled models that have become the norm over the last couple of decades. Minimalists say that lower, lighter models allow you to run with better, more natural form once you've adjusted to them. Many experienced runners find that running in a variety of shoes, including some minimalist models, is better than doing all of their running in the same shoes.

## N

**NEGATIVE SPLITS:** Running the second half of a race faster than the first half.

## O

**ORTHOTICS:** Devices worn inside running shoes to help treat or prevent injuries. Orthotics can be hard or soft and of varying length, depending on what injury they're trying to address. You should wear orthotics only if advised to by a sports medicine professional who says you need one to address a specific underlying imbalance or weakness.

**OUT-AND-BACK:** A course that entails running out to a turnaround spot, then running back to the starting point. Out-and-backs are a convenient way to get in runs in unfamiliar locales. They're also a good option when you're trying to run a little farther than you have before, because you don't have the option of cutting the run short.

**OVERUSE INJURY:** Any injury incurred from doing too much mileage before the body is ready. Examples of common overuse injuries among runners include runner's knee, iliotibial (IT) band syndrome, and plantar fasciitis.

**OVERPRONATION:** Excessive inward roll of the foot, which can cause pain in the foot, shin, and knee.

**OVERTRAINING:** A collapse in performance that occurs when the body gets pushed beyond its capacity to recover. It can lead to fatigue, stale training, poor race performance, irritability, and loss of enthusiasm for running.

Serious overtraining can cause sleep disturbances, hampered immune function, poor appetite, and the cessation of menstrual periods in women.

## P

**PACE:** How fast you're running, usually expressed in terms of minutes per mile. Your running pace at a given effort level will vary greatly from day to day, depending on the weather, your fatigue level, and numerous other factors. While it's good to have a general idea of how fast you're running, it's best not to base your running on hitting certain paces all the time. Doing so usually leads to working too hard and can drain much of the enjoyment from your running. As you gain fitness, you'll naturally speed up.

**PERSONAL RECORD (PR):** Term used to describe a runner's farthest or fastest time in a race. Also called a personal best (PB).

**PLANTAR FASCIA:** Thick connective tissue that runs along the bottom of your foot from the heel bone to the base of your toe bones. It can easily be inflamed by many of the same things that irritate the Achilles tendon, including too-rapid increases in distance and/or intensity and poor flexibility of the calf muscles.

## Q

**QUADS/QUADRICEPS:** The four main muscles in the front of your legs. They help to stabilize your knees after your foot hits the ground when you're running. New runners whose lives involve a lot of sitting often have tighter and shorter quad muscles than are ideal for running. Good quad strength and flexibility helps to relieve strain on your knees.

**QUALITY WORKOUTS:** Any workouts that are faster or longer than daily runs. Within the context of marathon and half-marathon training, the term usually refers to workouts such as long runs, speed sessions, and tempo runs, which all require a day or two of recovery.

## R

**RECOVERY:** Walking or easy jogging between faster-paced segments. Recovery lets your heart rate return to the point where you're ready to run fast again, and it helps you regain the energy you'll need for the next burst of speed.

**REPEATS:** The fast segments of running that are repeated during a workout, with recovery in between. If you're training for a marathon, you might run 1000-meter repeats six times. For shorter races, like 5-Ks, you might do shorter repeats of 400 meters or so at your goal race pace.

**RICE:** Refers to Rest, Ice, Compression, and Elevation. These measures can relieve pain, reduce swelling, and protect damaged tissues, all of which speed healing. They're most effective when done immediately following an injury. RICE is the standard prescription for many aches and pains, such as strained hamstrings and twisted ankles.

**RUN/WALK:** Method popularized by Olympian Jeff Galloway, columnist and author of *Runner's World*'s monthly "Starting Line" column. Walk breaks allow a runner to feel strong to the end and recover fast, while providing the same stamina and conditioning as a continuous run. By shifting back and forth between walking and running, you work a variety of different muscle groups, which helps fend off fatigue. To receive the maximum benefit, you must start the walk breaks before you feel any fatigue, during the first mile. If you wait until you feel the need for a walk break, then you've already let yourself get fatigued and defeated the purpose of the walk break.

**RUNNER'S KNEE:** A common running injury marked by inflammation of the underside of the kneecap. A common cause in new runners is building up mileage too quickly. Being at a good running weight and having strong, flexible quad and hip muscles help to lessen your risk for developing runner's knee.

## S

**SIDE STITCH:** Also called a "side sticker," this is a sharp pain usually felt just below the rib cage (though sometimes farther up the torso). It's thought to be caused by a cramp in the diaphragm, gas in the intestines, or food in the stomach. Stitches normally come on during hard workouts or races. To get rid of a side stitch, notice which foot is striking the ground when you inhale and exhale, then switch the pattern. So if you were leading with your right foot, inhale when your left foot steps. If that doesn't help, stop running and reach both arms above your head. Bend at your waist, leaning to the side opposite the stitch until the pain subsides.

**SPECIFICITY:** Training should be relevant and appropriate to the sport for which you're training in order to maximize performance. Long runs, for instance, as opposed to cycling, are specific training for marathons and half-marathons because they prepare your muscles for the specific activity that you'll be doing during the race: covering a long distance for hours at a time.

**SPEEDWORK:** Also called intervals or repeats, speedwork refers to any workout run at a faster-than-normal pace. Often done at a track. Performed to increase cardiovascular fitness.

**SPLITS:** The time it takes to complete any defined distance. If you're running 800 meters, or two laps, you might check your split after the first lap to shoot for an even pace.

**STREAKER:** Typically refers to someone who has completed a race multiple years in a row.

**STRIDE RATE:** The number of times your feet hit the ground during a minute of running. This measurement is often used to assess running efficiency. Having a high stride rate—say 170 steps per minute or more—can reduce injuries and help you run faster. Typically the number used refers to the total number of times either foot hits the ground. So for a person with a stride rate of 170, the right foot and the left foot would each have hit the ground 85 times.

**STRIDES:** Also called striders or "pickups," these are typically 80- to 100-meter surges that are incorporated into a warmup or a regular workout. Strides increase heart rate and leg turnover; they get your legs ready to run. Strides are run near 80 percent of maximum effort, with easy jogging in between.

**SUPINATION:** The insufficient inward roll of the foot after landing. This places extra stress on the foot and can result in iliotibial (IT) band syndrome, Achilles tendinitis, and plantar fasciitis. Runners with high arches and tight Achilles tendons tend to supinate.

# T

**TALK TEST:** A way to see if you're running at a comfortable effort level. During most of your runs, you should be able to carry on a conversation, which means you've passed the talk test. If you can't say more than a few words at a time, you're probably running too hard. Back off to where you can say a sentence at a time, and you'll be able to run longer and better advance your fitness.

**TECHNICAL CLOTHING:** This typically refers to clothing made of synthetic fibers that wick moisture away from the skin. These fibers do not absorb moisture like cotton does, and they help prevent uncomfortable chafing.

**TEMPO:** When runners talk about doing a "tempo run," they usually mean a sustained, faster-than-usual run of 3 to 6 miles at the pace they could sustain for an hour in a race. Tempo runs are said to feel "comfortably hard"—you have to concentrate to keep the effort going but aren't running with as much effort as a sprint or 5-K race. Tempo runs are a good way to boost your fitness without doing hard track workouts.

**10-K:** A race that's 6.2 miles long. Most runners cover the distance at least 15 seconds per mile slower than they do a 5-K.

**TEN PERCENT RULE:** Don't increase mileage or intensity by more than 10 percent from one week to another. This is a classic injury-prevention rule meant to prevent a runner from doing too much, too soon, and getting injured.

**TRACK:** Most tracks are 400 meters long. Four laps, or 1600 meters, is approximately equivalent to 1 mile. Many runners use the term "track" to refer to a speed session done on a track.

**TRAIL RUNNING:** Doing some or all of a run off-road. Trail running has become increasingly popular in part because running in the woods or mountains is usually more appealing than sharing the road with distracted drivers. Trails' softer surfaces are also a nice change from asphalt. Expect to run slower than usual on trails.

## U

**USATF:** USA Track & Field (usatf.org), the governing body of track and field, long-distance running, and race walking in the United States. This nonprofit organization selects and leads Team USA to compete at the Olympics, the World Championships, and other international events each year. It also certifies racecourses for accuracy, validates records, and establishes and enforces rules and regulations of the sport.

**ULTRA/ULTRAMARATHON:** Any race that's longer than a marathon. The most popular ultra distances are 50-K (31 miles), 50 miles, and 100-K (62 miles). A lot of ultras are run on trails or in other natural settings, and almost all ultras have much smaller fields than the average half-marathon or marathon.

## V

**$VO_2$ MAX:** A measurement of the maximum amount of oxygen that a person can consume per minute while exercising. $VO_2$ max is determined by genetics, gender, body composition, age, and training. Runners with a naturally high $VO_2$ max often find it easier to run faster because their hearts can deliver more oxygen to their muscles. There are many ways to boost $VO_2$ max, including speedwork, which forces the heart to pump blood at a higher rate.

## W

**WARMUP:** A period of walking or easy running or any light activity that is done for 10 to 20 minutes before a workout. It gradually increases heart rate, breathing rate, and blood flow to the muscles, and it prepares the body for more vigorous work. A good warmup allows the body to work more efficiently and helps prevent muscle pulls and strains.

**THE WALL:** Typically refers to a point when a runner's energy levels plummet, breathing becomes labored, and negative thoughts begin to flood in; this often happens at mile 20 of a marathon. Experts say that it usually happens two-thirds of the way through any race, no matter the distance. Hitting the wall often occurs because you've run out of fuel and need carbohydrates (like a sports drink or an energy gel) that the body can convert into fuel for the muscles to use.

**WIND CHILL:** How cold it really feels when you're outside. As the wind grows stronger, it feels much colder than the air temperature.

# NEED MOTIVATION? START RIGHT HERE.

**IN YOUR LOG,** write down details about how long and how far you went on each workout and how you felt while you were on the road. You'll draw confidence from seeing all of your workouts add up. And the next day's workout won't seem as intimidating when you see how much you've already accomplished.

**IN YOUR FIRST** few weeks, establish a workout routine that blends well into the rhythm of your daily life. Figure out what times of day are most convenient to work out, and find a variety of safe, traffic-free routes that you can take on a regular basis.

**THE IDEA OF** "starting an exercise routine" can seem daunting. It doesn't have to be. Begin with a 15-minute walk. Feeling good? The next day, do it again. If you're feeling strong, add 5 or 10 more minutes. Work up to 35 minutes by the end of the week.

**WORKING OUT** should push you out of your comfort zone, but training should never feel like torture. Find some way to work out that feels like fun to you. Run in a scenic area with friends you enjoy. Take a detour from your regular route to see streets you've never seen before. Get some new music or books to listen to on the go; or if you always tune in, try a tech-free run. Hit the gym, or get a friend or family member to join you on the road.

**FIND A BUDDY** to work out with or join a group workout or class. Studies have shown that connecting with others—whether it's in person or even through an online forum—boosts your chances of sticking with your exercise routine. You're less likely to blow off a workout when you know that someone is waiting for you. And you won't be as intimidated and self-conscious if you have company.

**THE PROSPECT** of PRs and weight loss can be overwhelming. Just focus on making good decisions one moment at a time.

**WHAT'S THE BEST** time of day to work out? It's whatever time of day you're most likely to actually get it done! Whether you're a morning person, a night owl, or someone who looks forward to a midday break to split up the workday, what matters most is clearing the roadblocks that get between you and your workout.

**PREP FOR AN** early-morning walk or run the night before. Set your automatic coffeemaker to brew before you wake. Turn off the computer and TV at least 30 minutes before you hit the sack, and get blackout shades for your windows—the absence of light boosts production of melatonin, a hormone that makes you feel sleepy. Move your alarm clock across the room, so you'll have to get out of bed to turn it off. And once you're up, put on your exercise clothes in a brightly lit room: When light hits your eyes, it signals your pineal gland to stop producing melatonin, helping you wake up.

**PLANNING A MIDDAY** workout? Schedule your walk or run like you would any other meeting; put it on your to-do list, and cross it off for the confidence boost that comes from mission accomplished. Split your lunch in two: Eat half of it an hour before you go out, then have the remaining food afterward. Don't stress about missing work—exercise has been proven to increase work productivity.

**PLANNING A LATE-DAY** workout? When you're mentally and physically tired at the end of the day, dopamine, the brain chemical that energizes you and makes you feel up, is going to be low, as is your blood sugar. But a good workout will energize you. Walking and running elevate your heart rate and nervous system, which will make you feel more alert. Pack your gear, change at work, and go directly to the gym or the trail. Keep your energy up with a snack before you exercise.

**EQUIP YOUR RUNNING** routine with the activities that will make you feel good about it and get you revved up to get up and go each day. Meet up with friends so that the run doubles as socializing time; track your miles so that you can see the progress you're making and the fitness improvements.

Connect with other runners online to share and celebrate your successes.

**USE A TRAINING** plan as a guide, but don't hesitate to swap workouts around to fit them into your busy schedule. While longer sessions are ideal, if you'd like to split up the workouts into two or three sessions at first, that's okay. Studies have shown that you get the same benefits from three 10-minute sessions as a single 30-minute workout.

**TUNING OUT**—not in—can help you get through those tough first workouts, says Christy Greenleaf, PhD, a professor of kinesiology at the University of Wisconsin. Recruit a friend to walk the neighborhood with you; watch your favorite sitcom while you're on the treadmill; put together a workout mix with tunes that evoke happy memories. "Any way that you can focus your attention on something other than how your body feels will help," says Greenleaf.

**WINTER CAN BE** a challenging time to stick to an exercise routine, and not just because of the weather. Aside from the ice, slush, snow, and far fewer hours of daylight to get those workouts in, you have to juggle it with holiday and family commitments. Exercising with a friend even once a week can help you get out the door, as it's harder to blow off a workout if you know that someone is waiting for you. And you don't necessarily have to run or walk. Making dates to lift weights at the gym or take a yoga or Pilates class can help you stay on track with these activities.

**STUDIES HAVE SHOWN** that about two-thirds of the way through any race, whatever the distance, runners tend to hit the wall. At that point, the excitement of the start has worn off, and the finish still feels like it's very far away. Anticipate that you're going to hit this tough stretch, and prepare for it. Break the distance down into segments. Just focus on running to the next block or lamppost. Once you get there, pick another target just ahead.

**FEEL TIRED?** Ease off to a pace where you can maintain a conversation; you should feel relaxed, like you could run at that pace for an entire day if you had to. If you're huffing and puffing, you're going too fast.

**MANY PEOPLE ARE** surprised to find that when they start exercising, the pounds don't just magically and immediately melt off. Whether you're ravenous when you return from your run, or you just feel entitled to treats, it's easy to go overboard. It's easy to eat back the calories you burned and then some. To avoid that, track your calorie intake with one of the many Web sites or apps; it will force you to pause and think before you taste, and exercise portion control. Also, schedule a nonfood reward when you reach certain milestones; some new running duds, a new book or some new music, a day at the spa, or a night out with friends.

**IF YOU START** to feel discouraged on the run, replay the "highlight reel" of the greatest moments of your life. In a training log, keep a running tally of the number of miles and time that you've spent working out so you always know how much you've accomplished. It will make whatever distance you still have to cover seem much more manageable.

**REMEMBER THAT JUST** by being out there, you're inspiring others who are still on the couch, and everyone who is driving by, and showing them what's possible. Keep moving.

**DON'T HESITATE TO** listen to music while you work out. Studies have shown that listening to music reduces the level of perceived exertion, or how hard you feel like you're working. But if you're running outside, be sure to use just one earbud so that you can hear oncoming traffic.

**REMEMBER: A SINGLE** workout won't make or break your fitness; it's the accumulated impact of fitness that you've built over the course of weeks or months that gets you in shape. But if you try to cram in miles in too short a period of time, you could get sidelined for weeks or months.

**WHILE EXERCISE IS** a proven stress reliever, if you start your workout frazzled or drained from your nonrunning life—say you are sick, sleep deprived, anxious about work, or you've been partying too hard—the workout is going to feel harder.

Studies have shown that for stressed-out people, workouts felt harder than for those who weren't stressed, even when they were working at the same effort level. Muscles also took longer to recover.

**AS YOU GET** fitter, it's especially important that you take good notes on your training, detailing how far and fast you went, how you felt while you were out, the terrain, the route, and what the weather conditions were. A well-kept log will help you fend off injuries: If you see that your knee was achy a few days in a row, you'll know to take a break before it becomes a full-blown injury.

**THOUGH IT SEEMS** like runners are everywhere, finding someone you want to work out with again and again can be tricky. Be prepared to ask direct questions about schedules, needs, and goals. Next to pace, possibly the most important factor is being able to meet at a mutually convenient time and place—even if that's side-by-side treadmills at the gym.

**EVERYONE HAS A** threshold for what's manageable, and you can get overwhelmed juggling work and family life. Be mindful of your own threshold. If winter is your least flexible time, don't sign up for a race that will require major time and energy commitments. Pick a more flexible time of year.

**SET MULTIPLE GOALS.** That way, if you miss your big goal, you have others that are still within reach. Develop process goals that aren't tied to outcome of a race or your runs. Instead of just focusing on doing a race, or reaching a target weight, aim to not slow down in the final miles of a run, or eliminate your walk breaks. These goals can be easier to achieve, which will give you a taste of success.

**IN THE EUPHORIA** of meeting someone who might be a good running mate, it's easy to commit to a long-term relationship. But it's a good idea to go for a few test runs before you promise more. You can go on a "first date" with a person without committing to a long-term training plan together.

**DON'T SLACK ON** your training log; it will help you avoid burnout. Say you're starting to feel bored and less motivated to get on the road. You might see in your log that you've taken the same 5-mile route for 3 months. You'll know it's time for a change.

**DEFINITELY CELEBRATE** your successes. But rather than rewarding yourself with food—even if it's sugar free, fat free, or calorie free—pat yourself on the back with something lasting and nonedible. Get a pedicure, buy a new outfit, meet up with friends, or get a new book or some new tunes.

**RUNNING WITH A** partner is one of the best ways to ensure that you get out the door for every workout. But your workout may unravel if you (a) talk so much that your pace slows to a crawl or (b) race each other until someone bonks. Remember why you're there: to boost your fitness and enjoy the camaraderie and support of one another.

**ANYTIME YOU'RE PUSHING** your body farther than it's gone before, focus on finishing feeling strong, not your finishing time. Once you go the distance, you can focus on building your speed.

**IF YOU DON'T** have a great workout or race, remind yourself of all the positive things running gives you—better health, stress relief, and opportunity to spend time in nature and bond with friends. Keeping those big-picture benefits on your radar can give you the motivation you need to keep pushing.

**INCORPORATING YOUR DOG** into your exercise regime can be a great way to stay consistent and get some quality together time. In fact, studies have shown that people who exercise with a dog are more likely to stick with it than those who go it alone or with a human partner. Be sure to start slow. If you're just starting to run, chances are your dog is too. Keep in mind that the dog's muscles, bones, and joints may need just as much time to adapt to your new routine as you do. Start with short distances and build gradually, just as you do to avoid injuries of your own.

**WHAT MAKES A GOOD** mantra? One that's short, positive, instructive, and full of action words. Prepare multiple mantras for different challenges you might encounter. It should address what you want to feel, not the adversity you're trying to overcome. Keep it to 5 seconds or less. Look for words that convey energy, like "fast," "strong," or "power."

**GROUP RUNS CAN** be a great way to mix social life and fitness. Most running shops have regular workouts, and you can find groups near you through local chapters of the Road Runners Club of America (RRCA.org) or sites like dailymile.com.

**BEFORE YOU JOIN** a group for the first time, get familiar with the route. To avoid getting lost, find out about the course the group will take when you join them. Drive it beforehand if possible.

**IF SOMEONE INVITES** you for a workout, do not bring an iPod with you. Enjoy the camaraderie and chance to talk!

**IF YOU'RE RUNNING** on a path, it's just like driving—always stick to the right-hand side.

**SET SHORT, ACHIEVABLE** goals. Break down your aspirations into daily, weekly, and monthly goals.

**WHENEVER YOU'RE IN** doubt, remember these wise words from *Runner's World* chief running officer Bart Yasso: "I often hear someone say, 'I'm not a real runner.' We are all runners; some just run faster than others. I never met a fake runner."

**YOU DON'T HAVE** to race to be a serious runner, but there are many good reasons to enter races. You get a sense of community from races. They help you realize that you belong to something big, and that more people than you imagined share your fitness goals.

**YOU WANT TO GET** something done? Do it early in the day. Everything gets tougher later in the day when various tasks and responsibilities start ganging up on you. In a recent *Runner's World Online* survey, the two most popular workout times were 5 a.m. and 6 a.m.

**ALWAYS HAVE A** complete bag of running gear (and a dry shirt and towel) at the ready in the trunk of your car. You never know when you'll be able to use them.

**SEE HOW MANY** different surfaces you can run on in a week: asphalt, gravel, trail, grass, track, treadmill, beach. Each stresses your leg muscles in a slightly different way, helping to prevent overuse injuries. (If possible, avoid concrete, the hardest and least-accommodating surface for runners.)

**IF YOU CAN'T** run in the morning or at lunchtime, at least try to run before you get home from work. Stop at a favorite park or trail on your way home from the office and do a workout there. Or arrange to meet some friends for a run at 5:30 p.m. Once you're at home, it's hard to get out the door again for a workout.

**SOMETIMES THE MOST** motivating and rewarding thing you can do is to reach out to someone else. It could be someone close: at work or even in your family. Or your club might receive occasional calls from new runners, or those who want to begin. Offer to help. Beginners don't need a mentor with a PhD. They need encouragement, a personal connection, and the kind of basic training, nutrition, and injury prevention experience you already possess.

**MANY RUNNING WEB SITES,** including ours, have forums or message boards where runners exchange information, opinions, and greetings that develop into digital friendships. Often these blossom into "encounters," where the online friends agree to meet at a particular race. Along the way, they encourage each other's training and lend a sympathetic ear when that's what they need most.

**YOU WISH EVERY DAY** will go as planned and every run will fit perfectly into the scheme of things. But stuff happens. Don't worry about the runs you miss. Sometimes the best advice is simply to run with a smile on your face, and to enjoy every workout. Come to think of it, that's always the best advice.

**RACE WEEK ISN'T** the time to try new shoes, new food or drinks, new gear, or anything else you haven't used on several workouts. Stick with the routine that works for you.

**5-KS AND 10-KS** are hugely positive community events. You get to spend a morning with strangers cheering you on, feeding you and offering water, and celebrating doing something healthy for yourself. Everyone fears that they'll be last, but don't worry. In all likelihood, you won't be. People with a very wide range of abilities and levels of fitness do 5-Ks, and many people just walk them from start to finish.

# NOTES